LOW FODMAP DIET COOKBOOK

1000 DAYS OF TASTY AND EASY RECIPES | ESSENTIAL GUIDE TO MANAGING IBS AND OTHER DIGESTIVE DISORDERS WITH A COMPREHENSIVE 58-DAY MEAL PLAN

SUSAN SINIARD

TABLE OF CONTENTS

Scan the QR Code and access your 3 bonuses in digital format

🔥 **Bonus 1: Dining Out Low FODMAP Guide**

🔥 **Bonus 2: Stress Management for IBS Relief**

🔥 **Bonus 3: The Ultimate Low FODMAP Shopping List**

CHAPTER 1

THE SCIENCE OF IBS AND FODMAPS

Irritable Bowel Syndrome (IBS) affects millions worldwide, manifesting in symptoms like bloating, abdominal pain, and altered bowel habits. Despite its prevalence, effective management remains elusive for many. Enter the Low FODMAP Diet, a scientifically backed approach that has revolutionized the treatment of IBS.

Developed through rigorous research, this diet significantly reduces symptoms by limiting foods high in certain fermentable carbohydrates known as FODMAPs. These compounds can trigger digestive distress in sensitive individuals and challenge daily activities. Understanding how to navigate this diet can transform lives, offering relief and a renewed sense of control. This guide delves deep into the nuances of IBS and the principles behind the low-FODMAPS diet, shedding light on the complex interactions between food and the gut.

Exploring the scientific foundation and practical application of this dietary strategy aims to empower readers with the knowledge and tools needed to reclaim their health and well-being. Here, you'll find not just a diet but a pathway to a better quality of life, underscored by the testimonies of those who have successfully completed this journey.

What is Irritable Bowel Syndrome (IBS)?

Living with IBS can be an ongoing journey of managing symptoms and understanding personal triggers, but advancements in both the knowledge and treatment of the syndrome continue to improve the quality of life for those affected. One of the more recent and significant shifts in managing IBS includes personalized dietary recommendations based on individual tolerance levels. The Low FODMAP diet, specifically designed to minimize the intake of certain carbohydrates poorly absorbed by the small intestine, has emerged as a pivotal strategy in controlling symptoms. This diet necessitates the elimination of various foods, including certain fruits, vegetables, grains, and dairy products, which are known to produce significant amounts of gas and osmotic pressure, thus exacerbating IBS symptoms.

Additionally, psychological therapies have proven effective for many dealing with IBS. Cognitive-behavioral therapy (CBT), for instance, helps patients develop strategies to manage the psychological stressors that may trigger gastrointestinal symptoms. Similarly, hypnotherapy has been used to reduce pain and improve the psychological well-being of IBS sufferers, with some studies showing improvements in over 50% of patients undergoing such treatments.

The establishment of a solid patient-provider connection is another essential component in managing IBS. Good communication between the patient and the healthcare practitioner is crucial because it enables treatment plans to be continuously modified in response to the patient's changing symptoms and way of life. Because it encourages patients to participate in their treatment actively, this dynamic approach can greatly enhance results by giving patients a greater sense of control over their condition.

Online forums and support groups are also very important for offering IBS sufferers both practical guidance and emotional support. These platforms offer a space for sharing experiences and solutions that have worked for others, helping to alleviate the feeling of isolation that many with IBS experience. Additionally, these communities can serve as a valuable resource for new research and dietary tips, which are particularly important given the ever-evolving nature of nutritional science related to gut health.

For many, the journey to managing IBS effectively is marked by periods of trial and error. The value of a customized strategy is highlighted by the possibility that what works for one individual may not work for another.

This individual variability can be frustrating; however, with persistence and the right support, many people find strategies that significantly mitigate their symptoms. It is also crucial for individuals with IBS to stay informed about new treatments and dietary practices as ongoing research continues to shed light on the complex interactions between diet, gut microbiota, and the immune system.

As research progresses, the hope is that more targeted therapies will emerge, offering more definitive relief and, perhaps, one day, a cure. Until then, the emphasis remains on managing symptoms to enhance the quality of life for those with IBS. This involves not only medical interventions and dietary adjustments but also understanding and accommodating personal and social environments that support individuals in managing their condition.

IBS can be a challenging and often unpredictable condition; the development of a comprehensive management plan tailored to the individual's specific symptoms and lifestyle can lead to significant improvements. By combining dietary strategies like the Low FODMAP diet with medical treatments, psychological support, and lifestyle modifications, those with IBS can achieve a better quality of life. As awareness grows and research advances, the prospects for effectively managing and one day eradicating IBS look increasingly promising. Through patient education, supportive communities, and ongoing medical research, there is hope for those affected by this often, debilitating condition.

The Scientific Discovery of FODMAPs

The journey to understand and manage Irritable Bowel Syndrome (IBS) and similar gastrointestinal disorders took a significant leap forward with the scientific discovery of FODMAPs. This discovery has not only revolutionized the dietary management of IBS but has also shed light on how certain foods can trigger digestive symptoms in sensitive individuals.

Fermentable Oligosaccharides, Disaccharides, Monosaccharides, and Polyols are short-chain carbohydrates and sugar alcohols that are poorly absorbed by the small intestine. The acronym "FODMAPS" itself refers to these substances.

The story of FODMAPs began in the late 1990s and early 2000s when researchers at Monash University in Australia started to delve deeper into the causes of IBS symptoms. The team, led by Dr. Peter Gibson and Dr. Susan Shepherd, was initially puzzled by the persistent digestive distress experienced by patients who appeared to be eating a healthy diet. Traditional wisdom at the time suggested that fiber was beneficial for gut health, yet many high-fiber foods seemed to exacerbate symptoms in certain individuals.

Through meticulous research, the Monash team discovered that while some foods high in fiber were indeed beneficial, others contained types of carbohydrates that were not well absorbed in the small intestine. This malabsorption led to fermentation by bacteria in the gut, producing gas and attracting water, which then caused bloating, gas, abdominal pain, and other symptoms associated with IBS.

To investigate this further, the researchers conducted controlled dietary trials, meticulously observing how patients responded to foods that were high and low in these specific carbohydrates. Their findings confirmed that diets high in these poorly absorbed sugars significantly increased symptoms of IBS, while diets low in these sugars (low-FODMAP diets) provided considerable relief. This was a groundbreaking discovery because it offered a new, non-pharmacological treatment for a condition that affects millions worldwide.

The fact that a large range of foods, including grains, sweets, fruits, and vegetables, contain FODMAPs makes them important. Typical examples include dairy items like milk and yogurt (lactose), apples and honey (fructose), onions and garlic (fructans), and sweeteners like sorbitol and mannitol. By knowing which foods are rich in fermentable sugars

(FODMAPS), people with IBS may adjust their diet to consume less of these fermentable sugars, which will help them manage their symptoms more successfully.

The implications of this research are profound. For one, it provides a clear and actionable strategy for managing IBS through diet, which can significantly improve the quality of life for many patients. It also helps to reduce the reliance on medications, which can carry side effects and often provide only symptomatic relief rather than addressing the root cause of the discomfort.

Furthermore, the research on FODMAPs has opened up a new field of gastrointestinal health, leading to further studies on how diet affects the gut microbiome—the complex community of microorganisms living in the digestive tracts. This is important since new research indicates that the gut microbiota is important for maintaining general health and preventing illness.

The low-FODMAP diet, developed based on this research, is now internationally recognized and recommended by healthcare providers worldwide for managing IBS symptoms. It has been adapted into various guidelines and resources to help patients understand and implement the diet in their lives. This includes detailed food lists, meal plans, and even smartphone apps designed to make following a low-FODMAP diet easier.

Educating patients about FODMAPs involves more than just providing lists of foods to avoid. It also includes training them on how to read food labels, understand food preparation and cooking processes that can affect FODMAP levels, and guide them on how to reintroduce foods to determine personal tolerance levels. This educational approach empowers patients, giving them control over their symptoms and reducing the fear and anxiety that often come with digestive health issues.

The ongoing research into FODMAPs continues to refine our understanding of gastrointestinal health. Scientists are now investigating the long-term impacts of the low-FODMAP diet on the gut microbiome and exploring potential modifications to the diet that might offer even greater benefits. Not only can this research help people with IBS, but it may also help those with other digestive problems, including celiac disease and inflammatory bowel disease (IBD).

The discovery of FODMAPs has been a pivotal moment in the field of digestive health. It has provided a scientific basis for dietary management of IBS, transforming the lives of many who suffer from this condition. As research continues, our understanding of FODMAPs and their role in diet and health will deepen, continuing to improve the strategies available for managing gastrointestinal disorders.

The Principles of Low FODMAP Eating

The low-FODMAPS diet offers a calculated method of controlling Irritable Bowel Syndrome (IBS) symptoms by cutting back on certain carbs that are known to cause pain. Understanding the foundational principles of this diet and how it interacts with the body to mitigate symptoms is essential for anyone looking to adopt it effectively.

At the core of the low FODMAP diet is the reduction of fermentable oligosaccharides, disaccharides, monosaccharides, and polyols— carbohydrates that are poorly absorbed in the small intestine. These carbohydrates are frequently included in a broad range of meals, such as wheat-based goods, dairy products high in lactose, fruits like apples and pears, and vegetables like onions and garlic. When these fermentable materials are eaten, bacteria in the stomach ferment them, which may cause the formation of more fluid and gas. This procedure typically results in the symptoms of IBS, which include bloating, gas, stomach pain, and changes in bowel patterns.

The low-FODMAPS diet follows a planned method that usually starts with the elimination phase, during which all items rich in FODMAPS are cut out of the diet. This phase is crucial for clearing the slate, so to speak, allowing both the patient and healthcare provider to identify specific triggers. During this time, many individuals experience a notable reduction in their symptoms, providing a clearer baseline from which to evaluate potential dietary triggers.

Following the initial elimination, the reintroduction phase begins, where one FODMAP group at a time is systematically reintroduced into the diet. This careful, methodical process is designed to identify which specific FODMAPs trigger symptoms and to what extent each individual can tolerate them without experiencing discomfort. This phase is integral as it helps to personalize the diet to the individual individual's specific needs, avoiding unnecessary restrictions and ensuring a more balanced, nutritionally adequate intake.

The final maintenance phase of the diet involves the continued avoidance of identified triggers while maintaining a balanced diet. This phase is intended to be a long-term solution that manages symptoms while still allowing for a varied and enjoyable diet. The goal here is to integrate this approach into a sustainable lifestyle that supports digestive health and overall well-being.

The effectiveness of the low FODMAP diet in managing IBS symptoms is supported by numerous studies, which show significant improvements in symptom severity and quality of life for many patients. The diet'sdiet's role extends beyond simple symptom management; it empowers individuals to understand the links between their diet and digestive health, fostering a sense of control over their condition.

Moreover, this diet emphasizes the importance of professional guidance. Due to its complex nature and the risk of nutritional deficiencies, navigating the low FODMAP diet should ideally be done under the supervision of a healthcare professional, particularly a dietitian specializing in gastrointestinal disorders. This ensures that the diet is followed correctly and that all nutritional needs are met.

The broader significance of the low FODMAP diet lies in its holistic impact on patients' lives. By reducing gastrointestinal symptoms, individuals often experience improvements in social interactions, mental health, and overall quality of life. The diet's effectiveness can decrease the anxiety associated with symptom flare-ups, particularly in social settings where food is involved.

The psychological benefit is also notable, as the diet reduces the stress and unpredictability associated with IBS. Having a clear plan that effectively manages symptoms can provide mental and emotional relief, which is just as important as physical relief. This aspect of the diet underscores the interconnectedness of physical health and mental well-being, highlighting the need for comprehensive treatment approaches that address both aspects.

Regarding education, the low-FODMAPS diet is an effective means of promoting knowledge regarding digestive health and the role that food plays in controlling long-term illnesses. It can be a gateway to broader discussions about the impact of nutrition on health, encouraging more research and a better understanding of gastrointestinal diseases.

The principles of low FODMAP eating provide a well-defined and effective framework for managing IBS symptoms. Through the elimination, reintroduction, and personalization phases, individuals can identify specific dietary triggers and develop a tailored eating plan that minimizes symptoms while maintaining nutritional balance. Supported by scientific research and clinical success, the low FODMAP diet stands as a testament to the power of diet in controlling chronic health conditions, offering renewed hope and improved quality of life to those affected by IBS.

Benefits and Challenges of the Diet

The low FODMAP diet heralded as a significant advancement in the management of Irritable Bowel Syndrome (IBS) and other related gastrointestinal conditions, offers a promising approach for those suffering from these often debilitating disorders. While the benefits of this dietary intervention can be substantial, implementing and maintaining the diet poses various challenges. Understanding both the advantages and hurdles can help individuals navigate the low FODMAP journey more effectively.

Benefits of the Low FODMAP Diet

One of the primary benefits of the low FODMAP diet is the alleviation of symptoms associated with IBS, which include abdominal pain, bloating, gas, diarrhea, and constipation. By significantly reducing the intake of foods high in fermentable carbohydrates, individuals often experience a marked decrease in these symptoms. This improvement can lead to enhanced quality of life, as the discomfort and stress associated with IBS symptoms are reduced.

Additionally, the diet promotes a more mindful approach to eating. Individuals become more aware of their food choices, learning to identify ingredients that might trigger symptoms. This heightened awareness can contribute to better long-term dietary habits and a deeper understanding of how food affects the body.

The low FODMAP diet also empowers individuals to regain control over their health. Many people with IBS experience frustration and helplessness due to the unpredictable nature of their symptoms. Through the structured approach of eliminating and reintroducing foods, individuals can pinpoint specific dietary triggers, allowing for more personalized and effective management of their condition.

Moreover, the positive changes in gastrointestinal symptoms often lead to improvements in overall well-being. Pain and discomfort can be reduced, which can improve mood and energy levels, lessen the anxiety associated with digestive problems, and facilitate social contacts and activities that were previously avoided out of concern about flare-ups of symptoms.

Challenges of the Low FODMAP Diet

Despite its effectiveness, the low FODMAP diet is challenging. One of the main difficulties is the initial phase of the diet, which involves strict avoidance of a broad range of foods. This restriction can be daunting and overwhelming, especially for those who are accustomed to a less restrictive diet.

A major obstacle may also come from the diet's intricacy. FODMAPs are present in high concentrations in many everyday meals, and recognizing them without the right information can be challenging. Misinformation and the subtleties of portion sizes can further complicate adherence to the diet.

The social repercussions of adhering to a tight diet provide another difficulty. Going out to eat, going to social events, and even having meals with your family might cause stress since it can be challenging to locate low-FODMAPS foods that are acceptable. Feelings of marginalization or loneliness may result from this.

In addition, improper food management increases the risk of nutritional deficiencies. Large categories of fruits, vegetables, grains, and dairy products should not be excluded since this may result in an insufficient diet of vitamins, fiber, and calcium, among other vital elements.

Overcoming the Challenges

Several strategies can be adopted to implement and sustain the low FODMAP diet successfully. Firstly, seeking guidance from a dietitian specialized in FODMAPs is crucial. These professionals can provide education on the diet, help plan meals, and ensure nutritional balance is maintained.

Education is key. Understanding which foods are low in FODMAPs, learning to read labels, and knowing how to substitute high FODMAP ingredients with low FODMAP alternatives can all alleviate much of the stress associated with the diet.

Gradual implementation may also ease the transition. Instead of overhauling the diet overnight, gradually reducing high FODMAP foods can help the body adjust without feeling overwhelmed.

For social situations, planning ahead is vital. Checking restaurant menus in advance, explaining dietary restrictions to hosts, or bringing own low FODMAP dishes to gatherings can help maintain social connections and reduce anxiety.

To address the risk of nutritional deficiencies, a balanced intake of low-FODMAP fruits, vegetables, grains, and alternative sources of calcium and fiber should be emphasized. Supplements may also be taken into consideration while working with a healthcare professional.

Lastly, staying informed about the latest FODMAP research and resources can provide ongoing support and motivation. Participating in online or live support groups can provide extra guidance and motivation from like-minded individuals.

The low FODMAP diet presents several challenges, but the benefits can be life-changing for individuals struggling with IBS and other gastrointestinal disorders. With the appropriate techniques and assistance, individuals following a low-FODMAPS diet may enhance their quality of life, successfully manage their symptoms, and take back control of their health.

How FODMAPs Affect the Gut

The group of carbohydrates known as FODMAPs, or fermentable oligosaccharides, disaccharides, monosaccharides, and polyols, is known to cause pain in certain people, especially those who have Irritable Bowel Syndrome (IBS). To fully appreciate how these substances affect the gut, it's crucial to understand their biological impact on the gastrointestinal tract and their interactions with the gut microbiome.

When FODMAPs are consumed, they enter the small intestine, where they are not absorbed effectively. Due to their small size and water-attracting nature, these carbohydrates draw water into the small intestine. This increase in fluid can result in diarrhea for some individuals, as the gut struggles to manage the sudden influx of water. For others, the presence of unabsorbed carbohydrates moving into the large intestine can lead to different issues.

In the large intestine, FODMAPs become food for the resident bacteria—a process known as fermentation. This fermentation can produce several types of gas, including hydrogen, methane, and carbon dioxide. The production of these gases can cause a range of symptoms associated with IBS, such as bloating, abdominal pain, and an altered bowel schedule, which can manifest as either constipation or diarrhea. The degree and type of symptomatology often depend on the types of gases produced and how the individual's body reacts to these gases.

The interaction of FODMAPs with the gut microbiome is particularly complex. The gut microbiome consists of a vast array of bacteria that play significant roles in health and disease. These microbes help digest food, protect against pathogens, and produce essential nutrients and neurotransmitters. When FODMAPs are fermented by these bacteria, it not only leads to gas production but can also influence the composition of the microbiome itself.

Research suggests that diets high in FODMAPs can alter the gut microbiome's composition, promoting the growth of bacteria that produce more gas and potentially reducing the prevalence of beneficial bacteria. This shift in the microbial population can exacerbate gastrointestinal symptoms and may impact the overall health of the gut. For example, the creation of short-chain fatty acids, which are essential for colon health and aid in regulating inflammation and cellular development, might be decreased by a decline in beneficial bacteria.

Moreover, a disorder called small intestinal bacterial overgrowth (SIBO), in which an excessive number of bacteria colonize the small intestine, might result from the quick fermentation of FODMAPs. SIBO often exacerbates the symptoms of IBS, leading to significant discomfort. Managing FODMAP intake can help control SIBO, reduce symptoms, and promote a healthier balance of intestinal bacteria.

The response to FODMAPs is highly individualized, influenced by the unique composition of each person's microbiome. Because of this individual diversity, dietary therapies such as the low-FODMAPS diet have the potential to be very successful. The diet limits the amount of these fermentable carbohydrates consumed, which lowers the substrate available for fermentation and, in turn, limits the generation of gas and the symptoms that go along with it.

Implementing a low FODMAP diet also often leads to changes in the gut microbiome. Initially, this might involve a reduction in the diversity of the microbiome, as some bacteria starve from the lack of fermentable carbohydrates. However, many individuals find that with careful management and strategic reintroduction of certain carbohydrates, they can maintain a balanced and healthy microbiome while also keeping their symptoms in check.

It's essential for individuals following a low FODMAP diet to do so under professional guidance to ensure that they achieve a nutritional balance and do not unduly restrict their intake of essential nutrients. Dietitians can help tailor the diet to include a variety of foods that support gut health and promote a robust microbiome, such as introducing permissible quantities of prebiotics that nourish beneficial bacteria.

The study of FODMAPs and their impact on the gut is a growing field that continues to reveal how critical diet is to managing gastrointestinal health. The understanding that emerges not only helps those with IBS manage their symptoms more effectively but also enhances the broader knowledge of gut health. This insight into the relationship between diet, the gut microbiome, and overall health underscores the importance of a thoughtful, personalized approach to nutrition—one that respects the complexity of the human body and the variability among individuals.

FODMAPs play a significant role in gut health by affecting biological processes in the gastrointestinal tract and interacting with the gut microbiome. Managing the intake of these carbohydrates can significantly reduce IBS symptoms and promote a healthier gut environment, demonstrating the profound impact of diet on our well-being.

CHAPTER 2

PREPARING FOR THE LOW FODMAP JOURNEY

Embarking on the low FODMAP diet is a decisive step towards managing digestive discomfort and enhancing overall gut health. This journey requires careful planning and commitment, as it involves understanding which foods to avoid and which to embrace to alleviate symptoms associated with Irritable Bowel Syndrome (IBS) and other related conditions. Essential to this process is the preparation of one's kitchen and pantry, ensuring that all high-FODMAP foods are replaced with suitable alternatives that do not trigger symptoms.

Additionally, adopting the right cooking techniques can make a substantial difference in successfully maintaining a low FODMAP diet. This dietary change isn't only about avoiding particular foods for those with chronic digestive problems; it's also about making well-considered decisions that may significantly enhance quality of life. The initial efforts in organizing and preparing for this diet pave the way for smoother transitions, making daily meal planning less daunting and more intuitive. As such, setting the stage with the right tools and knowledge is crucial for anyone ready to start their low FODMAP journey.

The Essential Low FODMAP Pantry

Setting up your pantry when following a low FODMAP diet is essential to ensure you have the right ingredients on hand for meals that won't trigger your symptoms. Here's a detailed guide to building a pantry that supports your low FODMAP lifestyle, complete with essential items and tips for avoiding high FODMAP foods.

Grains are fundamental to a balanced diet, and for those following a low FODMAP diet, certain grains are preferable. Rice, both white and brown, is a versatile and safe choice, providing a comforting base for a variety of dishes. Oats are another excellent option for breakfast, while quinoa offers a protein-packed alternative suitable for salads, sides, or even as a main component of a meal. Additionally, look for gluten-free pasta made from rice or corn, which can help diversify your meal options without causing discomfort.

Navigating sweeteners can be tricky on a low FODMAP diet. Many common sweeteners, like honey and high fructose corn syrup, are high in FODMAPs and can trigger symptoms. Safe alternatives include pure maple syrup and regular table sugar, both of which can be used to sweeten everything from baked goods to coffee without adverse effects.

Canned goods can be particularly useful for those on a restricted diet, providing convenience and extended shelf life. Look for canned chickpeas and lentils, which are low in FODMAPs when rinsed thoroughly before use. Plain canned tomatoes are also a staple for creating low FODMAP sauces and stews; just be sure they don't contain added high FODMAP ingredients like onion or garlic.

When it comes to snacks, nuts and seeds are nutritious options that fit well within a low FODMAP diet. Walnuts, macadamia nuts, peanuts, and pumpkin seeds are all safe choices in moderation. However, it's important to be mindful of portion sizes, as eating too much of any nut can lead to increased FODMAP intake and potential symptoms.

Condiments and spices can add flavor to your meals without adding FODMAPs if chosen carefully. Mustard, mayonnaise, and gluten-free soy sauce are all safe options that can enhance the taste of your dishes. When using spices and herbs, opt for pure forms without added fillers or flavors that could contain high FODMAP ingredients.

For those who consume dairy or its alternatives, lactose-free milk and hard cheeses are generally well-tolerated. Plant-based milk alternatives like almond milk and rice milk are also good choices, provided they don't contain additives like inulin, which is high in FODMAPs.

Reading labels is critical when shopping for low-FODMAP ingredients. Always scan the ingredient list for hidden FODMAPs such as inulin, wheat, onion, garlic, and stone fruits. Ingredients are listed by weight, so even if a high FODMAP ingredient is listed at the end, its smaller proportion might not trigger symptoms, though it's always safer to avoid these ingredients entirely if possible.

Utilizing resources such as low FODMAP food lists and smartphone apps can also be incredibly helpful. These tools provide up-to-date information on which foods are safe and which should be avoided, making it easier to shop and plan meals confidently.

Building a low FODMAP pantry doesn't mean you have to give up flavor or variety in your diet. By choosing the right ingredients and learning to navigate food labels effectively, you can enjoy delicious, varied meals that won't compromise your digestive health. Over time, these habits will become second nature, and managing your diet will feel more like a routine part of life rather than a daily challenge.

With a well-stocked low FODMAP pantry, the stress of managing digestive symptoms becomes much more manageable. This preparation allows for creativity in the kitchen, enabling you to explore new recipes and cuisines that keep your meals exciting and satisfying. Whether you're cooking a simple weekday dinner or preparing a special meal for friends and family, having the right ingredients at your fingertips is the key to a successful and enjoyable low-FODMAP diet experience.

Tools and Techniques for Low FODMAP Cooking

Embracing a low FODMAP diet can transform the way you approach cooking and eating, especially if you suffer from IBS or similar gastrointestinal issues. Successfully managing this diet is easier with the right kitchen tools and cooking techniques that minimize the presence of high FODMAP ingredients while maximizing flavor and nutritional value.

When setting up your kitchen for low FODMAP cooking, several essential tools can make the process smoother and more enjoyable. A good set of knives is indispensable, as much of the diet revolves around fresh, whole ingredients that need to be precisely chopped, diced, or sliced. A durable cutting board is also necessary, and having several boards can help prevent cross-contamination, especially if you share your kitchen with others who are not following a low FODMAP diet.

Measuring cups and spoons are crucial for managing portion sizes, which is vital for ingredients that can be tolerated in small amounts but may trigger symptoms in larger quantities. Digital scales help ensure that your measurements are accurate, supporting effective management of FODMAP intake.

Blenders and food processors are invaluable tools in a low FODMAP kitchen. They allow you to make smoothies, soups, and sauces that are free of high FODMAP ingredients like onions and garlic. For instance, blending a base of tomatoes, carrots, and herbs can produce a flavorful sauce without the need for traditional but high FODMAP additives.

Non-stick cookware can also be a game-changer, reducing the need for excessive amounts of oil, which can be helpful since some individuals with digestive issues also experience difficulties processing fats. With a good quality non-stick skillet or pan, you can sauté vegetables and meats without fear of sticking, using just a small amount of garlic-infused oil— a low FODMAP alternative to whole garlic—to enhance flavor without triggering symptoms.

In addition to having the right tools, adopting specific cooking techniques can further help maintain a low FODMAP diet. Steaming is a particularly effective method, ideal for cooking vegetables and fish. It preserves nutrients and natural flavors without using any high FODMAP ingredients. Steaming can be done with a simple metal or bamboo steamer over a pot of boiling water. This technique is excellent for preparing delicate foods like spinach, zucchini, and carrots, which are low FODMAP-friendly at certain serving sizes.

Slow cooking is another technique well-suited for low FODMAP recipes. Using a slow cooker allows for the development of deep, rich flavors over several hours, which is perfect for cooking meats and whole grains like rice or quinoa. You can create hearty, satisfying dishes such as stews and casseroles, which are easy to digest and low in FODMAPs, provided you carefully choose the ingredients according to low FODMAP guidelines.

Fermentation is a traditional technique that can be adapted for low FODMAP cooking. While many fermented foods are high in FODMAPs, homemade recipes can be adjusted to fit the diet. For example, fermenting your own yogurts using lactose-free milk or creating fermented vegetables without the use of garlic or onions can be beneficial. These provide the gut-friendly benefits of fermented foods while keeping FODMAP levels in check.

Roasting is another useful technique, perfect for enhancing the natural sweetness and flavor of low FODMAP vegetables like potatoes, carrots, and bell peppers. A light drizzle of garlic-infused oil and a sprinkle of safe herbs and spices before roasting can turn these simple ingredients into a delicious, gut-friendly side dish.

Lastly, mastering the art of flavor enhancement without high FODMAP ingredients is crucial. Utilizing herbs and spices such as basil, parsley, thyme, and ginger can add layers of flavor to your dishes without adding FODMAPs. Experimenting with infused oils, like the garlic-infused oil mentioned earlier, along with chives and scallions (green parts only), can also introduce onion and garlic flavors safely.

While following a low-FODMAPS diet may seem like a cooking restriction at first, with the correct equipment and methods, it may open up new culinary possibilities and help you find a diet that not only improves your symptoms but also satisfies your taste buds. This method of cooking not only improves the health of your digestive system but also your entire well-being by enabling you to eat tasty, healthy meals without worrying about being uncomfortable.

CHAPTER 3

RECIPES

Embarking on a low FODMAP diet doesn't mean sacrificing flavor or diversity in your meals. With the right recipes, you can enjoy a wide array of delicious dishes that cater to your dietary needs while still being satisfying and enjoyable. Cooking within these guidelines offers an opportunity to explore a variety of ingredients and cooking techniques, ensuring that meals are not only safe for your gut but also appealing to the palate. Whether you're craving hearty breakfasts, nourishing lunches, or sumptuous dinners, the possibilities are endless. Each recipe has been crafted to ensure it fits within the low FODMAP parameters, using ingredients that minimize the risk of digestive discomfort. This section provides a collection of recipes designed to bring joy and variety back to your dining table, proving that a diet tailored to gastrointestinal health can be rich, varied, and incredibly tasty. These recipes, which range from salads and smoothies to entrees and sweets, will support the daily maintenance of a healthy, balanced diet.

Breakfast (25 Recipes)

Sunrise Smoothie with Banana and Strawberry

Ingredients:

- 1 ripe banana
- 1 cup strawberries, hulled
- 1/2 cup lactose-free yogurt
- 1/2 cup almond milk
- 1 tablespoon chia seeds
- 1 teaspoon honey (optional)

Directions:

1. Combine the banana, strawberries, lactose-free yogurt, almond milk, and chia seeds in a blender.
2. Blend until smooth.
3. Taste and add honey if desired.
4. Pour into a glass and enjoy immediately.

Nutritional Values (per serving):

- Calories: 180
- Fat: 4g
- Carbohydrates: 34g
- Protein: 6g

Blueberry Infused Quinoa Porridge

Ingredients:

- 1 cup quinoa, rinsed
- 2 cups water
- 1 cup lactose-free milk
- 1/2 cup blueberries
- 1 tablespoon maple syrup
- 1/2 teaspoon vanilla extract
- 1/4 teaspoon ground cinnamon

Directions:

1. In a medium saucepan, bring quinoa and water to a boil.
2. Reduce heat to low, cover, and simmer for 15 minutes.
3. Stir in lactose-free milk, blueberries, maple syrup, vanilla extract, and cinnamon.
4. Cook for another 5-10 minutes, stirring occasionally, until thick and creamy.
5. Serve warm, garnished with additional blueberries if desired.

Nutritional Values (per serving):

- Calories: 220

- Fat: 4g
- Carbohydrates: 38g
- Protein: 7g

Spinach and Feta Omelet

Ingredients:

- 3 large eggs
- 1/4 cup lactose-free milk
- 1/2 cup fresh spinach, chopped
- 1/4 cup crumbled feta cheese
- 1 tablespoon olive oil
- Salt and pepper to taste

Directions:

1. In a bowl, whisk together the eggs and lactose-free milk until well combined.
2. Heat olive oil in a non-stick skillet over medium heat.
3. Add spinach and sauté until wilted.
4. Pour the egg mixture into the skillet and cook until the edges start to set.
5. Sprinkle feta cheese evenly over the omelet.
6. Fold the omelet in half and continue cooking until fully set.
7. Season with salt and pepper before serving.

Nutritional Values (per serving):

- Calories: 250
- Fat: 20g
- Carbohydrates: 3g
- Protein: 15g

Cinnamon Buckwheat Pancakes

Ingredients:

- 1 cup buckwheat flour
- 1 tablespoon baking powder
- 1/2 teaspoon ground cinnamon
- 1 cup lactose-free milk
- 1 large egg
- 2 tablespoons maple syrup
- 1 tablespoon olive oil
- 1 teaspoon vanilla extract

Directions:

1. In a large bowl, whisk together the buckwheat flour, baking powder, and cinnamon.
2. In another bowl, mix the lactose-free milk, egg, maple syrup, olive oil, and vanilla extract.
3. Combine the wet and dry ingredients, stirring until just combined.

4. Heat a non-stick skillet over medium heat and lightly grease with oil.

5. Pour 1/4 cup of batter onto the skillet and cook until bubbles form on the surface, then flip and cook until golden brown.

6. Repeat with the remaining batter.

7. Serve warm with additional maple syrup if desired.

Nutritional Values (per serving):

- Calories: 210
- Fat: 8g
- Carbohydrates: 30g
- Protein: 6g

Maple-Glazed Chicken Sausage Patties

Ingredients:

- 1 pound ground chicken
- 1/4 cup pure maple syrup
- 1/2 teaspoon ground sage
- 1/2 teaspoon ground thyme
- 1/2 teaspoon salt
- 1/4 teaspoon black pepper
- 1 tablespoon olive oil

Directions:

1. In a bowl, combine the ground chicken, maple syrup, sage, thyme, salt, and pepper. Mix well.

2. Form the mixture into small patties.

3. Heat olive oil in a large skillet over medium heat.

4. Cook the patties for 5-6 minutes on each side, or until golden brown and cooked through.

5. Serve warm, drizzled with a little extra maple syrup if desired.

Nutritional Values (per serving):

- Calories: 180
- Fat: 8g
- Carbohydrates: 6g
- Protein: 20g

Low FODMAP Muesli with Oats and Seeds

Ingredients:

- 2 cups rolled oats
- 1/2 cup pumpkin seeds
- 1/2 cup sunflower seeds
- 1/4 cup shredded coconut

- 1/4 cup dried cranberries (ensure they are low FODMAP)
- 1 teaspoon ground cinnamon
- 1/2 teaspoon vanilla extract

Directions:

1. In a large bowl, combine rolled oats, pumpkin seeds, sunflower seeds, shredded coconut, and dried cranberries.
2. Add ground cinnamon and vanilla extract, mixing well.
3. Store in an airtight container.
4. Serve with lactose-free milk or yogurt.

Nutritional Values (per serving):

- Calories: 250
- Fat: 12g
- Carbohydrates: 30g
- Protein: 7g

Lactose-Free Yogurt Parfait with Kiwi

Ingredients:

- 1 cup lactose-free yogurt
- 1 kiwi, peeled and sliced
- 1/4 cup low FODMAP granola
- 1 tablespoon chia seeds

Directions:

1. In a glass or bowl, layer half of the lactose-free yogurt.
2. Add a layer of sliced kiwi.
3. Sprinkle with low FODMAP granola and chia seeds.
4. Repeat the layers with the remaining ingredients.
5. Serve immediately.

Nutritional Values (per serving):

- Calories: 200
- Fat: 6g
- Carbohydrates: 30g
- Protein: 10g

Sweet Potato and Bacon Hash

Ingredients:

- 2 large sweet potatoes, peeled and diced
- 4 strips of bacon, chopped
- 1 bell pepper, diced
- 1/2 cup chopped green onions (green parts only)
- 1 tablespoon olive oil
- Salt and pepper to taste

Directions:

1. In a large skillet, cook bacon over medium heat until crispy. Remove and set aside, leaving the bacon fat in the skillet.

2. Add olive oil to the skillet and heat over medium-high heat.

3. Add sweet potatoes and cook for 10-15 minutes, until tender and slightly crispy.

4. Stir in bell pepper and cook for an additional 5 minutes.

5. Add green onions and cooked bacon, stirring to combine.

6. Season with salt and pepper before serving.

Nutritional Values (per serving):

- Calories: 250
- Fat: 10g
- Carbohydrates: 35g
- Protein: 6g

Raspberry Chia Pudding

Ingredients:

- 1 cup lactose-free milk
- 1/4 cup chia seeds
- 1/2 cup fresh raspberries
- 1 tablespoon maple syrup
- 1/2 teaspoon vanilla extract

Directions:

1. In a bowl, combine lactose-free milk, chia seeds, maple syrup, and vanilla extract.

2. Stir well and let sit for 10 minutes. Stir again to prevent clumping.

3. Refrigerate for at least 4 hours, or overnight.

4. Before serving, mash half of the raspberries and mix into the pudding.

5. Top with remaining raspberries.

Nutritional Values (per serving):

- Calories: 200
- Fat: 8g
- Carbohydrates: 25g
- Protein: 5g

Spiced Pumpkin Waffles

Ingredients:

- 1 cup pumpkin puree
- 2 large eggs
- 1 cup lactose-free milk
- 1 tablespoon olive oil
- 1 cup gluten-free flour
- 1 tablespoon baking powder
- 1 teaspoon ground cinnamon
- 1/2 teaspoon ground ginger

- 1/4 teaspoon ground nutmeg
- 1/4 teaspoon salt

Directions:

1. In a large bowl, whisk together pumpkin puree, eggs, lactose-free milk, and olive oil.

2. In another bowl, mix gluten-free flour, baking powder, cinnamon, ginger, nutmeg, and salt.

3. Combine the wet and dry ingredients, stirring until just combined.

4. Preheat and lightly grease a waffle iron.

5. Pour batter into the waffle iron and cook according to the manufacturer's instructions until golden brown.

6. Serve warm with maple syrup or your favorite low FODMAP toppings.

Nutritional Values (per serving):

- Calories: 180
- Fat: 7g
- Carbohydrates: 25g
- Protein: 4g

Scrambled Tofu with Bell Peppers

Ingredients:

- 1 block firm tofu, drained and crumbled
- 1 red bell pepper, diced
- 1 green bell pepper, diced
- 1 tablespoon olive oil
- 1/2 teaspoon turmeric
- 1/4 teaspoon paprika
- Salt and pepper to taste
- 2 green onions (green parts only), chopped

Directions:

1. Heat olive oil in a large skillet over medium heat.

2. Add bell peppers and cook until tender, about 5 minutes.

3. Add crumbled tofu, turmeric, and paprika, stirring well.

4. Cook for another 5-7 minutes, until tofu is heated through and slightly crispy.

5. Season with salt and pepper.

6. Stir in chopped green onions before serving.

Nutritional Values (per serving):

- Calories: 220
- Fat: 12g
- Carbohydrates: 10g

- Protein: 18g

Ginger Pear Overnight Oats

Ingredients:

- 1 cup rolled oats
- 1 cup lactose-free milk
- 1 pear, diced
- 1 tablespoon chia seeds
- 1 teaspoon grated fresh ginger
- 1 tablespoon maple syrup

Directions:

1. In a bowl, combine rolled oats, lactose-free milk, diced pear, chia seeds, fresh ginger, and maple syrup.

2. Stir well to combine.

3. Cover and refrigerate overnight.

4. In the morning, give the oats a good stir and add a splash of lactose-free milk if needed to reach desired consistency.

5. Serve chilled.

Nutritional Values (per serving):

- Calories: 300
- Fat: 7g
- Carbohydrates: 50g

- Protein: 8g

FODMAP-friendly Eggs Benedict

Ingredients:

- 2 large eggs
- 2 slices gluten-free bread, toasted
- 1/2 avocado, sliced
- 2 tablespoons lactose-free yogurt
- 1 teaspoon lemon juice
- 1/2 teaspoon Dijon mustard
- Salt and pepper to taste
- Chopped chives for garnish

Directions:

1. Poach the eggs: Bring a pot of water to a gentle simmer and create a vortex. Crack eggs one at a time into the water and poach for 3-4 minutes until whites are set but yolks are still runny. Remove with a slotted spoon.

2. In a small bowl, mix lactose-free yogurt, lemon juice, Dijon mustard, salt, and pepper to create a quick hollandaise sauce.

3. Place avocado slices on the toasted gluten-free bread.

4. Top each slice with a poached egg.

5. Drizzle with the yogurt hollandaise sauce and garnish with chopped chives.

Nutritional Values (per serving):

- Calories: 320

- Fat: 18g

- Carbohydrates: 28g

- Protein: 12g

Turkey and Egg Breakfast Burrito

Ingredients:

- 1 gluten-free tortilla

- 2 large eggs

- 1/4 cup cooked turkey breast, diced

- 1/4 cup lactose-free cheese, shredded

- 1/4 avocado, sliced

- 1 tablespoon salsa (ensure it's low FODMAP)

- Salt and pepper to taste

- Olive oil for cooking

Directions:

1. In a skillet, heat a small amount of olive oil over medium heat.

2. Beat the eggs in a bowl, season with salt and pepper, and pour into the skillet. Scramble until cooked through.

3. Warm the gluten-free tortilla in another skillet or microwave.

4. Place scrambled eggs, diced turkey, shredded cheese, avocado slices, and salsa in the center of the tortilla.

5. Fold in the sides and roll up the burrito.

6. Serve warm.

Nutritional Values (per serving):

- Calories: 350

- Fat: 18g

- Carbohydrates: 28g

- Protein: 20g

Green Smoothie Bowl

Ingredients:

- 1 ripe banana, frozen

- 1 cup spinach

- 1/2 avocado

- 1/2 cup lactose-free milk

- 1 tablespoon chia seeds

- 1 tablespoon almond butter

- Toppings: fresh berries, coconut flakes, granola

Directions:

1. In a blender, combine the frozen banana, spinach, avocado, lactose-free milk, chia seeds, and almond butter.

2. Blend until smooth and thick.

3. Pour into a bowl and top with fresh berries, coconut flakes, and granola.

4. Serve immediately.

Nutritional Values (per serving):

- Calories: 300

- Fat: 15g

- Carbohydrates: 40g

- Protein: 7g

Strawberry Almond Muffins

Ingredients:

- 1 cup almond flour

- 1/2 cup gluten-free flour

- 1/2 teaspoon baking soda

- 1/4 teaspoon salt

- 2 large eggs

- 1/2 cup lactose-free yogurt

- 1/4 cup maple syrup

- 1 teaspoon vanilla extract

- 1 cup strawberries, diced

Directions:

1. Preheat the oven to 350°F (175°C) and line a muffin tin with paper liners.

2. In a large bowl, mix almond flour, gluten-free flour, baking soda, and salt.

3. In another bowl, whisk together eggs, lactose-free yogurt, maple syrup, and vanilla extract.

4. Combine the wet and dry ingredients, stirring until just combined.

5. Fold in the diced strawberries.

6. Divide the batter evenly among the muffin cups.

7. Bake for 20-25 minutes, or until a toothpick inserted into the center comes out clean.

8. Let cool before serving.

Nutritional Values (per serving):

- Calories: 180

- Fat: 9g

- Carbohydrates: 20g

- Protein: 5g

Baked Oatmeal with Blueberries

Ingredients:

- 2 cups rolled oats
- 1 teaspoon baking powder
- 1 teaspoon ground cinnamon
- 1/2 teaspoon salt
- 2 cups lactose-free milk
- 1 large egg
- 1/4 cup maple syrup
- 2 tablespoons melted coconut oil
- 1 teaspoon vanilla extract
- 1 cup fresh blueberries

Directions:

1. Preheat the oven to 375°F (190°C) and grease a baking dish.
2. In a large bowl, combine rolled oats, baking powder, cinnamon, and salt.
3. In another bowl, whisk together lactose-free milk, egg, maple syrup, melted coconut oil, and vanilla extract.
4. Pour the wet ingredients into the dry ingredients and mix well.
5. Gently fold in the blueberries.
6. Pour the mixture into the prepared baking dish.
7. Bake for 35-40 minutes, or until the top is golden brown and the oats are set.
8. Serve warm.

Nutritional Values (per serving):

- Calories: 220
- Fat: 8g
- Carbohydrates: 35g
- Protein: 6g

Quinoa Breakfast Bars

Ingredients:

- 2 cups cooked quinoa
- 1/2 cup almond butter
- 1/4 cup maple syrup
- 1/4 cup chia seeds
- 1/4 cup shredded coconut
- 1/2 cup dried cranberries (ensure they are low FODMAP)
- 1 teaspoon vanilla extract

Directions:

1. Preheat the oven to 350°F (175°C) and line a baking pan with parchment paper.
2. In a large bowl, mix cooked quinoa, almond butter, maple syrup, chia seeds, shredded coconut, dried cranberries, and

vanilla extract until well combined.

3. Press the mixture firmly into the prepared baking pan.

4. Bake for 20-25 minutes, or until the edges are golden brown.

5. Let cool completely before cutting into bars.

Nutritional Values (per serving):

- Calories: 200
- Fat: 10g
- Carbohydrates: 25g
- Protein: 5g

Lactose-Free Cottage Cheese with Pineapple

Ingredients:

- 1 cup lactose-free cottage cheese
- 1/2 cup fresh pineapple, diced
- 1 tablespoon chia seeds
- 1 teaspoon honey (optional)

Directions:

1. In a bowl, combine lactose-free cottage cheese, diced pineapple, and chia seeds.

2. Stir well to mix.

3. Drizzle with honey if desired.

4. Serve immediately.

Nutritional Values (per serving):

- Calories: 180
- Fat: 5g
- Carbohydrates: 20g
- Protein: 15g

Sourdough French Toast with Maple Syrup

Ingredients:

- 4 slices of sourdough bread
- 2 large eggs
- 1/2 cup lactose-free milk
- 1 teaspoon vanilla extract
- 1/2 teaspoon ground cinnamon
- 1 tablespoon butter
- Maple syrup for serving

Directions:

1. In a shallow bowl, whisk together eggs, lactose-free milk, vanilla extract, and ground cinnamon.

2. Heat a skillet over medium heat and add butter.

3. Dip each slice of sourdough bread into the egg mixture, coating both sides.

4. Place the coated bread slices in the skillet and cook until golden brown on both sides.

5. Serve warm with maple syrup.

Nutritional Values (per serving):

- Calories: 280
- Fat: 12g
- Carbohydrates: 32g
- Protein: 10g

Poached Eggs over Polenta

Ingredients:

- 2 cups water
- 1/2 cup polenta
- 1/4 cup grated Parmesan cheese
- 1 tablespoon butter
- 2 large eggs
- Salt and pepper to taste
- Chopped fresh herbs for garnish

Directions:

1. In a saucepan, bring water to a boil. Gradually whisk in the polenta.

2. Reduce heat to low and cook, stirring frequently, until thickened, about 15 minutes.

3. Stir in grated Parmesan cheese and butter. Season with salt and pepper.

4. Meanwhile, poach the eggs: bring a pot of water to a gentle simmer and create a vortex. Crack eggs one at a time into the water and poach for 3-4 minutes until whites are set but yolks are still runny. Remove with a slotted spoon.

5. Spoon the polenta onto plates and top each serving with a poached egg.

6. Garnish with chopped fresh herbs before serving.

Nutritional Values (per serving):

- Calories: 240
- Fat: 12g
- Carbohydrates: 20g
- Protein: 12g

Rice Cereal with Cinnamon Apples

Ingredients:

- 1 cup cooked rice
- 1 cup lactose-free milk
- 1 apple, peeled and diced
- 1 tablespoon maple syrup
- 1/2 teaspoon ground cinnamon

- 1/4 teaspoon vanilla extract

Directions:

1. In a saucepan, combine cooked rice, lactose-free milk, diced apple, maple syrup, ground cinnamon, and vanilla extract.

2. Cook over medium heat, stirring frequently, until the mixture is warm and the apples are tender.

3. Serve warm.

Nutritional Values (per serving):

- Calories: 220
- Fat: 3g
- Carbohydrates: 40g
- Protein: 5g

Turkey Sausage and Bell Pepper Skillet

Ingredients:

- 1 pound ground turkey
- 1 red bell pepper, diced
- 1 green bell pepper, diced
- 1 tablespoon olive oil
- 1 teaspoon dried oregano
- 1/2 teaspoon smoked paprika
- Salt and pepper to taste

Directions:

1. In a large skillet, heat olive oil over medium heat.

2. Add ground turkey and cook until browned, breaking it up with a spoon.

3. Add diced bell peppers, oregano, smoked paprika, salt, and pepper.

4. Cook until the bell peppers are tender and the turkey is cooked through.

5. Serve warm.

Nutritional Values (per serving):

- Calories: 200
- Fat: 10g
- Carbohydrates: 10g
- Protein: 20g

Oat and Banana Pancakes

Ingredients:

- 1 cup rolled oats
- 1 ripe banana
- 1 large egg
- 1/2 cup lactose-free milk
- 1 teaspoon vanilla extract
- 1/2 teaspoon baking powder
- 1/4 teaspoon ground cinnamon

Directions:

1. In a blender, combine rolled oats, banana, egg, lactose-free milk, vanilla extract, baking powder, and ground cinnamon.

2. Blend until smooth.

3. Heat a non-stick skillet over medium heat and lightly grease with oil.

4. Pour 1/4 cup of batter onto the skillet and cook until bubbles form on the surface, then flip and cook until golden brown.

5. Repeat with the remaining batter.

6. Serve warm with maple syrup or fresh fruit.

Nutritional Values (per serving):

- Calories: 180
- Fat: 5g
- Carbohydrates: 28g
- Protein: 5g

Zucchini and Carrot Fritters

Ingredients:

- 1 medium zucchini, grated
- 1 medium carrot, grated
- 1/4 cup gluten-free flour
- 1 large egg
- 1 tablespoon chopped fresh parsley
- 1/4 teaspoon ground cumin
- Salt and pepper to taste
- Olive oil for frying

Directions:

1. In a bowl, combine grated zucchini and carrot. Squeeze out excess moisture using a clean towel.

2. Add gluten-free flour, egg, parsley, cumin, salt, and pepper to the bowl. Mix well.

3. Heat olive oil in a large skillet over medium heat.

4. Drop spoon fuls of the mixture into the skillet and flatten slightly with a spatula.

5. Cook until golden brown on both sides, about 3-4 minutes per side.

6. Drain on paper towels and serve warm.

Nutritional Values (per serving):

- Calories: 150
- Fat: 8g
- Carbohydrates: 14g
- Protein: 4g

Lunch (25 Recipes)

Grilled Chicken Salad with Low FODMAP Vinaigrette

Ingredients:

- 2 boneless, skinless chicken breasts
- 4 cups mixed salad greens
- 1 cup cherry tomatoes, halved
- 1 cucumber, sliced
- 1/4 cup crumbled feta cheese
- 2 tablespoons olive oil
- 1 tablespoon red wine vinegar
- 1 teaspoon Dijon mustard
- Salt and pepper to taste

Directions:

1. Season chicken breasts with salt and pepper. Grill over medium heat for 6-7 minutes on each side, or until cooked through. Let rest and slice.

2. In a small bowl, whisk together olive oil, red wine vinegar, Dijon mustard, salt, and pepper to make the vinaigrette.

3. In a large bowl, combine mixed salad greens, cherry tomatoes, cucumber, and feta cheese.

4. Top with sliced grilled chicken and drizzle with vinaigrette.

5. Serve immediately.

Nutritional Values (per serving):

- Calories: 300
- Fat: 20g
- Carbohydrates: 10g
- Protein: 25g

Turkey and Swiss Cheese Wrap

Ingredients:

- 1 gluten-free tortilla
- 3 slices deli turkey breast
- 2 slices Swiss cheese
- 1/4 avocado, sliced
- 1 cup mixed greens
- 1 tablespoon mayonnaise (ensure it's low FODMAP)
- 1 teaspoon Dijon mustard

Directions:

1. Lay the gluten-free tortilla flat and spread with mayonnaise and Dijon mustard.

2. Layer turkey slices, Swiss cheese, avocado, and mixed greens on the tortilla.

3. Roll up the tortilla tightly.

4. Slice in half and serve.

Nutritional Values (per serving):

- Calories: 350

- Fat: 18g

- Carbohydrates: 28g

- Protein: 20g

Quinoa Tabbouleh with Cucumbers

Ingredients:

- 1 cup cooked quinoa

- 1 cucumber, diced

- 1/2 cup cherry tomatoes, halved

- 1/4 cup chopped fresh parsley

- 1/4 cup chopped fresh mint

- 2 tablespoons olive oil

- 1 tablespoon lemon juice

- Salt and pepper to taste

Directions:

1. In a large bowl, combine cooked quinoa, cucumber, cherry tomatoes, parsley, and mint.

2. In a small bowl, whisk together olive oil, lemon juice, salt, and pepper.

3. Pour the dressing over the quinoa mixture and toss to combine.

4. Serve chilled.

Nutritional Values (per serving):

- Calories: 220

- Fat: 10g

- Carbohydrates: 28g

- Protein: 5g

Low FODMAP Minestrone Soup

Ingredients:

- 2 tablespoons olive oil

- 1 carrot, diced

- 1 celery stalk, diced (green part only)

- 1 zucchini, diced

- 1 cup diced tomatoes (canned, no added garlic or onions)

- 4 cups low FODMAP vegetable broth

- 1/2 cup green beans, chopped

- 1/2 cup canned chickpeas, rinsed

- 1 teaspoon dried basil

- 1 teaspoon dried oregano
- Salt and pepper to taste

Directions:

1. In a large pot, heat olive oil over medium heat.

2. Add carrot, celery, and zucchini, and cook until tender, about 5 minutes.

3. Stir in diced tomatoes, vegetable broth, green beans, chickpeas, basil, and oregano.

4. Bring to a boil, then reduce heat and simmer for 20-25 minutes.

5. Season with salt and pepper before serving.

Nutritional Values (per serving):

- Calories: 150
- Fat: 7g
- Carbohydrates: 18g
- Protein: 5g

Baked Salmon with Herb Crust

Ingredients:

- 4 salmon fillets
- 1/4 cup gluten-free breadcrumbs
- 2 tablespoons chopped fresh parsley
- 2 tablespoons chopped fresh dill
- 1 tablespoon olive oil
- 1 teaspoon lemon zest
- Salt and pepper to taste

Directions:

1. Preheat the oven to 375°F (190°C).

2. In a small bowl, combine gluten-free breadcrumbs, parsley, dill, olive oil, lemon zest, salt, and pepper.

3. Place salmon fillets on a baking sheet lined with parchment paper.

4. Press the breadcrumb mixture onto the tops of the salmon fillets.

5. Bake for 15-20 minutes, or until the salmon is cooked through and the topping is golden brown.

6. Serve warm.

Nutritional Values (per serving):

- Calories: 300
- Fat: 18g
- Carbohydrates: 10g
- Protein: 28g

Rice Paper Rolls with Shrimp

Ingredients:

- 8 rice paper wrappers
- 16 cooked shrimp, peeled and deveined
- 1 cup shredded lettuce
- 1/2 cup shredded carrots
- 1/2 cup cucumber, julienned
- 1/4 cup fresh mint leaves
- 1/4 cup fresh basil leaves
- 1/4 cup fresh cilantro leaves
- 1/4 cup low FODMAP peanut sauce for dipping

Directions:

1. Soak one rice paper wrapper at a time in warm water for about 10-15 seconds until pliable.
2. Place the softened wrapper on a clean surface and arrange 2 shrimp, lettuce, carrots, cucumber, mint, basil, and cilantro in the center.
3. Fold the bottom of the wrapper over the filling, then fold in the sides and roll up tightly.
4. Repeat with remaining ingredients.
5. Serve with low FODMAP peanut sauce for dipping.

Nutritional Values (per serving):

- Calories: 120
- Fat: 2g
- Carbohydrates: 18g
- Protein: 10g

Greek Salad with Feta and Olives

Ingredients:

- 4 cups chopped romaine lettuce
- 1 cup cherry tomatoes, halved
- 1 cucumber, sliced
- 1/4 cup sliced black olives
- 1/4 cup crumbled feta cheese
- 2 tablespoons olive oil
- 1 tablespoon red wine vinegar
- 1 teaspoon dried oregano
- Salt and pepper to taste

Directions:

1. In a large bowl, combine romaine lettuce, cherry tomatoes, cucumber, olives, and feta cheese.
2. In a small bowl, whisk together olive oil, red wine vinegar, oregano, salt, and pepper.

3. Pour the dressing over the salad and toss to combine.

4. Serve immediately.

Nutritional Values (per serving):

- Calories: 180

- Fat: 14g

- Carbohydrates: 8g

- Protein: 5g

Sourdough Grilled Cheese with Spinach

Ingredients:

- 4 slices sourdough bread

- 2 tablespoons butter

- 1 cup fresh spinach

- 4 slices lactose-free cheese

Directions:

1. Butter one side of each slice of sourdough bread.

2. Heat a skillet over medium heat and add spinach, cooking until wilted.

3. Assemble sandwiches by placing cheese and cooked spinach between two slices of bread, buttered sides out.

4. Place the sandwiches in the skillet and cook until the bread is golden brown and the cheese

is melted, about 3-4 minutes per side.

5. Serve warm.

Nutritional Values (per serving):

- Calories: 320

- Fat: 20g

- Carbohydrates: 28g

- Protein: 12g

Tuna Salad Stuffed Bell Peppers

Ingredients:

- 2 bell peppers, halved and seeds removed

- 1 can tuna, drained

- 1/4 cup mayonnaise (ensure it's low FODMAP)

- 1 tablespoon lemon juice

- 1 tablespoon chopped fresh parsley

- Salt and pepper to taste

Directions:

1. In a bowl, combine tuna, mayonnaise, lemon juice, parsley, salt, and pepper.

2. Spoon the tuna mixture into the bell pepper halves.

3. Serve immediately or chill until ready to serve.

Nutritional Values (per serving):

- Calories: 200
- Fat: 12g
- Carbohydrates: 6g
- Protein: 18g

Vegetable Stir-fry with Ginger Sauce

Ingredients:

- 2 tablespoons olive oil
- 1 red bell pepper, sliced
- 1 yellow bell pepper, sliced
- 1 zucchini, sliced
- 1 cup snap peas
- 1 tablespoon grated fresh ginger
- 2 tablespoons low sodium soy sauce (gluten-free)
- 1 tablespoon rice vinegar
- 1 teaspoon sesame oil
- 1 teaspoon cornstarch mixed with 2 tablespoons water

Directions:

1. Heat olive oil in a large skillet or wok over medium-high heat.
2. Add bell peppers, zucchini, and snap peas, cooking until tender-crisp, about 5-7 minutes.
3. In a small bowl, whisk together grated ginger, soy sauce, rice vinegar, sesame oil, and cornstarch mixture.
4. Pour the sauce over the vegetables and stir to coat. Cook for another 2-3 minutes, until the sauce thickens.
5. Serve warm.

Nutritional Values (per serving):

- Calories: 150
- Fat: 7g
- Carbohydrates: 18g
- Protein: 4g

Chicken Caesar Salad (Lactose-Free Dressing)

Ingredients:

- 2 boneless, skinless chicken breasts
- 4 cups chopped romaine lettuce
- 1/4 cup lactose-free Parmesan cheese, grated
- 1/2 cup croutons (gluten-free)
- 1/4 cup mayonnaise (ensure it's low FODMAP)
- 1 tablespoon lemon juice
- 1 teaspoon Dijon mustard

- 1 teaspoon Worcestershire sauce (ensure it's low FODMAP)
- Salt and pepper to taste

Directions:

1. Season chicken breasts with salt and pepper. Grill over medium heat for 6-7 minutes on each side, or until cooked through. Let rest and slice.

2. In a small bowl, whisk together mayonnaise, lemon juice, Dijon mustard, Worcestershire sauce, salt, and pepper to make the dressing.

3. In a large bowl, combine romaine lettuce, grilled chicken slices, Parmesan cheese, and croutons.

4. Drizzle with dressing and toss to combine.

5. Serve immediately.

Nutritional Values (per serving):

- Calories: 350
- Fat: 20g
- Carbohydrates: 14g
- Protein: 30g

FODMAP-friendly Falafel Bowls

Ingredients:

- 1 can chickpeas, rinsed and drained
- 1/4 cup chopped fresh parsley
- 2 tablespoons flour (gluten-free)
- 1 tablespoon lemon juice
- 1 teaspoon ground cumin
- 1/2 teaspoon ground coriander
- Salt and pepper to taste
- 2 tablespoons olive oil
- 2 cups mixed salad greens
- 1/2 cup cherry tomatoes, halved
- 1/4 cup lactose-free tzatziki sauce (optional)

Directions:

1. In a food processor, combine chickpeas, parsley, flour, lemon juice, cumin, coriander, salt, and pepper. Pulse until the mixture is combined but still slightly chunky.

2. Form the mixture into small patties.

3. Heat olive oil in a large skillet over medium heat.

4. Cook the patties for 3-4 minutes on each side, until golden brown and crispy.

5. Serve the falafel over mixed salad greens with cherry tomatoes and a drizzle of tzatziki sauce if desired.

Nutritional Values (per serving):

- Calories: 300
- Fat: 15g
- Carbohydrates: 30g
- Protein: 10g

Turkey Meatballs with Gluten-Free Pasta

Ingredients:

- 1 pound ground turkey
- 1/4 cup gluten-free breadcrumbs
- 1/4 cup grated Parmesan cheese
- 1 egg
- 1 tablespoon chopped fresh parsley
- 1 teaspoon dried oregano
- Salt and pepper to taste
- 2 tablespoons olive oil
- 1 jar low FODMAP marinara sauce
- 8 ounces gluten-free pasta

Directions:

1. In a large bowl, combine ground turkey, gluten-free breadcrumbs, Parmesan cheese, egg, parsley, oregano, salt, and pepper. Mix well and form into meatballs.
2. Heat olive oil in a large skillet over medium heat.
3. Cook the meatballs until browned on all sides and cooked through, about 10-12 minutes.
4. Add marinara sauce to the skillet and simmer for 10 minutes.
5. Meanwhile, cook the gluten-free pasta according to package instructions.
6. Serve the meatballs and sauce over the cooked pasta.

Nutritional Values (per serving):

- Calories: 400
- Fat: 18g
- Carbohydrates: 35g
- Protein: 25g

Egg Salad on Gluten-Free Bread

Ingredients:

- 4 hard-boiled eggs, chopped

- 1/4 cup mayonnaise (ensure it's low FODMAP)

- 1 tablespoon Dijon mustard

- 1 tablespoon chopped fresh chives

- Salt and pepper to taste

- 4 slices gluten-free bread, toasted

Directions:

1. In a bowl, combine chopped eggs, mayonnaise, Dijon mustard, chives, salt, and pepper.

2. Mix until well combined.

3. Spread the egg salad on toasted gluten-free bread slices.

4. Serve immediately.

Nutritional Values (per serving):

- Calories: 300

- Fat: 20g

- Carbohydrates: 22g

- Protein: 10g

Roasted Vegetable and Quinoa Salad

Ingredients:

- 2 cups cooked quinoa

- 1 red bell pepper, diced

- 1 yellow bell pepper, diced

- 1 zucchini, diced

- 1 tablespoon olive oil

- 1/4 cup crumbled feta cheese

- 2 tablespoons chopped fresh parsley

- 1 tablespoon lemon juice

- Salt and pepper to taste

Directions:

1. Preheat the oven to 400°F (200°C).

2. Toss bell peppers and zucchini with olive oil, salt, and pepper. Spread on a baking sheet and roast for 20-25 minutes, until tender.

3. In a large bowl, combine cooked quinoa, roasted vegetables, feta cheese, parsley, and lemon juice.

4. Toss to combine and serve warm or chilled.

Nutritional Values (per serving):

- Calories: 250

- Fat: 10g

- Carbohydrates: 32g

- Protein: 8g

Beef and Spinach Stuffed Peppers

Ingredients:

- 4 bell peppers, tops cut off and seeds removed
- 1 pound ground beef
- 2 cups fresh spinach, chopped
- 1 cup cooked rice
- 1/2 cup tomato sauce (ensure it's low FODMAP)
- 1/4 cup grated Parmesan cheese
- 1 teaspoon dried oregano
- Salt and pepper to taste

Directions:

1. Preheat the oven to 375°F (190°C).
2. In a skillet, cook ground beef over medium heat until browned. Add spinach and cook until wilted.
3. In a large bowl, combine cooked beef and spinach, rice, tomato sauce, Parmesan cheese, oregano, salt, and pepper.
4. Stuff the mixture into the bell peppers and place them in a baking dish.
5. Cover with foil and bake for 30 minutes. Remove the foil and bake for an additional 10 minutes.
6. Serve warm.

Nutritional Values (per serving):

- Calories: 350
- Fat: 20g
- Carbohydrates: 20g
- Protein: 22g

Caprese Salad with Balsamic Glaze

Ingredients:

- 4 ripe tomatoes, sliced
- 8 ounces fresh mozzarella, sliced
- 1/4 cup fresh basil leaves
- 2 tablespoons olive oil
- 1 tablespoon balsamic glaze
- Salt and pepper to taste

Directions:

1. Arrange tomato slices, mozzarella slices, and basil leaves on a platter.
2. Drizzle with olive oil and balsamic glaze.
3. Season with salt and pepper before serving.

Nutritional Values (per serving):

- Calories: 250
- Fat: 18g
- Carbohydrates: 10g
- Protein: 12g

Lemon Herb Chicken Breast

Ingredients:

- 4 boneless, skinless chicken breasts
- 2 tablespoons olive oil
- 1 tablespoon lemon juice
- 1 teaspoon lemon zest
- 1 tablespoon chopped fresh rosemary
- 1 tablespoon chopped fresh thyme
- Salt and pepper to taste

Directions:

1. Preheat the oven to 375°F (190°C).
2. In a small bowl, combine olive oil, lemon juice, lemon zest, rosemary, thyme, salt, and pepper.
3. Place chicken breasts in a baking dish and brush with the lemon herb mixture.
4. Bake for 25-30 minutes, or until the chicken is cooked through.
5. Serve warm.

Nutritional Values (per serving):

- Calories: 280
- Fat: 12g
- Carbohydrates: 2g
- Protein: 38g

Lentil Soup with Carrots and Celery

Ingredients:

- 2 tablespoons olive oil
- 1 onion, diced (optional if sensitive)
- 2 carrots, diced
- 2 celery stalks, diced (green parts only)
- 1 cup dried lentils, rinsed
- 6 cups low FODMAP vegetable broth
- 1 teaspoon dried thyme
- 1 bay leaf
- Salt and pepper to taste

Directions:

1. In a large pot, heat olive oil over medium heat. Add onion

(if using), carrots, and celery, cooking until tender.

2. Stir in lentils, vegetable broth, thyme, and bay leaf.

3. Bring to a boil, then reduce heat and simmer for 30-35 minutes, or until lentils are tender.

4. Season with salt and pepper before serving.

Nutritional Values (per serving):

- Calories: 200
- Fat: 5g
- Carbohydrates: 30g
- Protein: 10g

Avocado and Shrimp Rice Bowl

Ingredients:

- 1 cup cooked rice
- 1/2 pound cooked shrimp, peeled and deveined
- 1 avocado, diced
- 1/2 cup diced cucumber
- 2 tablespoons chopped fresh cilantro
- 1 tablespoon lime juice
- 1 tablespoon olive oil
- Salt and pepper to taste

Directions:

1. In a bowl, combine cooked rice, shrimp, avocado, cucumber, and cilantro.

2. Drizzle with lime juice and olive oil.

3. Season with salt and pepper before serving.

Nutritional Values (per serving):

- Calories: 350
- Fat: 15g
- Carbohydrates: 30g
- Protein: 20g

Baked Haddock with Lemon and Dill

Ingredients:

- 4 haddock fillets
- 2 tablespoons olive oil
- 1 tablespoon lemon juice
- 1 teaspoon lemon zest
- 2 tablespoons chopped fresh dill
- Salt and pepper to taste

Directions:

1. Preheat the oven to 375°F (190°C).

2. Place haddock fillets in a baking dish.

3. In a small bowl, combine olive oil, lemon juice, lemon zest, dill, salt, and pepper.

4. Brush the mixture over the haddock fillets.

5. Bake for 15-20 minutes, or until the fish is cooked through and flakes easily with a fork.

6. Serve warm.

Nutritional Values (per serving):

- Calories: 220
- Fat: 10g
- Carbohydrates: 2g
- Protein: 30g

FODMAP-friendly Pad Thai

Ingredients:

- 8 ounces rice noodles
- 1/2 pound shrimp, peeled and deveined
- 2 tablespoons olive oil
- 2 eggs, beaten
- 1 cup bean sprouts
- 2 green onions (green parts only), chopped
- 1/4 cup chopped peanuts
- 1 tablespoon tamarind paste
- 2 tablespoons fish sauce
- 1 tablespoon lime juice
- 1 tablespoon brown sugar
- Fresh cilantro and lime wedges for garnish

Directions:

1. Cook rice noodles according to package instructions. Drain and set aside.

2. In a large skillet, heat olive oil over medium heat. Add shrimp and cook until pink, about 2-3 minutes per side. Remove and set aside.

3. Add beaten eggs to the skillet and scramble until cooked through. Remove and set aside with the shrimp.

4. In the same skillet, add bean sprouts and green onions, cooking for 2-3 minutes.

5. In a small bowl, whisk together tamarind paste, fish sauce, lime juice, and brown sugar.

6. Return noodles, shrimp, and eggs to the skillet. Pour the sauce over and toss to combine.

7. Serve with chopped peanuts, fresh cilantro, and lime wedges.

Nutritional Values (per serving):

- Calories: 400
- Fat: 18g
- Carbohydrates: 42g
- Protein: 20g

Zucchini Noodle Bowl with Pesto

Ingredients:

- 2 large zucchinis, spiralized into noodles
- 1/2 cup cherry tomatoes, halved
- 1/4 cup lactose-free feta cheese, crumbled
- 1/4 cup basil pesto (ensure it's low FODMAP)
- 1 tablespoon olive oil
- Salt and pepper to taste

Directions:

1. In a large skillet, heat olive oil over medium heat. Add zucchini noodles and cook for 3-4 minutes, until tender.
2. Add cherry tomatoes and cook for an additional 2 minutes.
3. Remove from heat and toss with basil pesto.
4. Top with crumbled feta cheese and season with salt and pepper before serving.

Nutritional Values (per serving):

- Calories: 250
- Fat: 20g
- Carbohydrates: 12g
- Protein: 6g

Smoked Salmon on Gluten-Free Crackers

Ingredients:

- 8 gluten-free crackers
- 4 ounces smoked salmon
- 1/4 cup lactose-free cream cheese
- 1 tablespoon capers
- 1 tablespoon chopped fresh dill
- Lemon wedges for garnish

Directions:

1. Spread lactose-free cream cheese on each gluten-free cracker.
2. Top with a slice of smoked salmon.
3. Garnish with capers and chopped dill.
4. Serve with lemon wedges.

Nutritional Values (per serving):

- Calories: 120
- Fat: 8g

- Carbohydrates: 8g
- Protein: 6g

Chicken and Rice Soup

Ingredients:

- 2 tablespoons olive oil
- 1 onion, diced (optional if sensitive)
- 2 carrots, diced
- 2 celery stalks, diced (green parts only)
- 1 pound boneless, skinless chicken breasts, cubed
- 1 cup cooked rice
- 6 cups low FODMAP chicken broth
- 1 bay leaf
- 1 teaspoon dried thyme
- Salt and pepper to taste

Directions:

1. In a large pot, heat olive oil over medium heat. Add onion (if using), carrots, and celery, cooking until tender.
2. Add cubed chicken and cook until no longer pink.
3. Stir in cooked rice, chicken broth, bay leaf, and thyme.
4. Bring to a boil, then reduce heat and simmer for 20-25 minutes.
5. Season with salt and pepper before serving.

Nutritional Values (per serving):

- Calories: 250
- Fat: 8g
- Carbohydrates: 20g
- Protein: 22g

Dinner (25 Recipes)

Maple-Glazed Pork Tenderloin

Ingredients:

- 1 pork tenderloin (about 1 pound)
- 1/4 cup pure maple syrup
- 2 tablespoons Dijon mustard
- 1 tablespoon olive oil
- 1 teaspoon dried thyme
- Salt and pepper to taste

Directions:

1. Preheat the oven to 375°F (190°C).
2. In a small bowl, mix maple syrup, Dijon mustard, olive oil, thyme, salt, and pepper.
3. Place the pork tenderloin in a baking dish and brush with the maple glaze.
4. Roast in the oven for 25-30 minutes, basting occasionally with the glaze, until the internal temperature reaches 145°F (63°C).
5. Let rest for 5 minutes before slicing.
6. Serve warm.

Nutritional Values (per serving):

- Calories: 250
- Fat: 10g
- Carbohydrates: 15g
- Protein: 25g

Baked Cod with Olive Tapenade

Ingredients:

- 4 cod fillets
- 1/2 cup black olives, pitted and chopped
- 1 tablespoon capers, drained
- 1 tablespoon olive oil
- 1 teaspoon lemon juice
- 1 teaspoon dried oregano
- Salt and pepper to taste

Directions:

1. Preheat the oven to 400°F (200°C).
2. In a small bowl, combine chopped olives, capers, olive oil, lemon juice, oregano, salt, and pepper.

3. Place cod fillets on a baking sheet lined with parchment paper.

4. Top each fillet with the olive tapenade mixture.

5. Bake for 12-15 minutes, or until the fish is cooked through and flakes easily with a fork.

6. Serve warm.

Nutritional Values (per serving):

- Calories: 180
- Fat: 8g
- Carbohydrates: 2g
- Protein: 24g

Spaghetti Squash with Tomato Sauce

Ingredients:

- 1 large spaghetti squash
- 2 tablespoons olive oil
- 1 can (14.5 ounces) diced tomatoes (no added garlic or onions)
- 1 teaspoon dried basil
- 1 teaspoon dried oregano
- Salt and pepper to taste
- 1/4 cup grated Parmesan cheese

Directions:

1. Preheat the oven to 375°F (190°C).

2. Cut the spaghetti squash in half lengthwise and remove the seeds.

3. Brush the cut sides with 1 tablespoon of olive oil and season with salt and pepper.

4. Place the squash halves cut side down on a baking sheet and bake for 40-45 minutes, until tender.

5. While the squash is baking, heat the remaining olive oil in a saucepan over medium heat. Add diced tomatoes, basil, oregano, salt, and pepper. Simmer for 10-15 minutes.

6. Scrape the flesh of the baked squash with a fork to create spaghetti-like strands. Toss with the tomato sauce and top with grated Parmesan cheese.

7. Serve warm.

Nutritional Values (per serving):

- Calories: 180
- Fat: 10g
- Carbohydrates: 18g
- Protein: 6g

Grilled Steak with Low FODMAP Chimichurri

Ingredients:

- 2 ribeye steaks
- Salt and pepper to taste
- 1/2 cup fresh parsley, chopped
- 1/4 cup fresh cilantro, chopped
- 2 tablespoons red wine vinegar
- 1/4 cup olive oil
- 1 teaspoon dried oregano
- 1/2 teaspoon crushed red pepper flakes

Directions:

1. Season steaks with salt and pepper.
2. Grill over medium-high heat for 4-5 minutes per side for medium-rare, or until desired doneness. Let rest.
3. In a small bowl, combine parsley, cilantro, red wine vinegar, olive oil, oregano, and red pepper flakes. Mix well.
4. Spoon chimichurri sauce over the steaks before serving.

Nutritional Values (per serving):

- Calories: 450
- Fat: 35g
- Carbohydrates: 2g
- Protein: 28g

Lemon Garlic Roasted Chicken

Ingredients:

- 1 whole chicken (about 4 pounds)
- 1/4 cup olive oil
- 2 tablespoons lemon juice
- 1 tablespoon lemon zest
- 1 tablespoon fresh thyme leaves
- 4 cloves garlic, minced (optional if sensitive)
- Salt and pepper to taste

Directions:

1. Preheat the oven to 375°F (190°C).
2. In a small bowl, combine olive oil, lemon juice, lemon zest, thyme, garlic (if using), salt, and pepper.
3. Rub the mixture all over the chicken, including under the skin.
4. Place the chicken in a roasting pan and roast for 1 hour and 15 minutes, or until the internal temperature reaches 165°F (74°C).
5. Let rest for 10 minutes before carving.

6. Serve warm.

Nutritional Values (per serving):

- Calories: 400

- Fat: 28g

- Carbohydrates: 2g

- Protein: 32g

Eggplant Parmesan (Gluten-Free)

Ingredients:

- 2 large eggplants, sliced into 1/2-inch rounds

- 1 cup gluten-free breadcrumbs

- 1/2 cup grated Parmesan cheese

- 2 eggs, beaten

- 2 cups marinara sauce (ensure it's low FODMAP)

- 1 cup shredded mozzarella cheese

- 1 tablespoon olive oil

- Salt and pepper to taste

Directions:

1. Preheat the oven to 375°F (190°C).

2. In a bowl, combine gluten-free breadcrumbs, Parmesan cheese, salt, and pepper.

3. Dip each eggplant slice in beaten egg, then coat with breadcrumb mixture.

4. Heat olive oil in a skillet over medium heat. Fry eggplant slices until golden brown on both sides.

5. In a baking dish, spread a layer of marinara sauce. Arrange eggplant slices on top, then add more sauce and sprinkle with mozzarella cheese.

6. Repeat layers, finishing with mozzarella cheese on top.

7. Bake for 25-30 minutes, or until the cheese is melted and bubbly.

8. Serve warm.

Nutritional Values (per serving):

- Calories: 300

- Fat: 18g

- Carbohydrates: 22g

- Protein: 12g

Moroccan Lamb Stew

Ingredients:

- 1 pound lamb shoulder, cubed

- 2 tablespoons olive oil

- 1 onion, diced (optional if sensitive)

- 2 carrots, diced
- 2 cups low FODMAP chicken broth
- 1 can (14.5 ounces) diced tomatoes (no added garlic or onions)
- 1/2 cup dried apricots, chopped
- 1 teaspoon ground cumin
- 1 teaspoon ground cinnamon
- 1 teaspoon ground ginger
- Salt and pepper to taste
- 1/4 cup chopped fresh cilantro

Directions:

1. In a large pot, heat olive oil over medium heat. Add lamb and cook until browned on all sides. Remove and set aside.

2. Add onion (if using) and carrots to the pot, cooking until tender.

3. Return lamb to the pot and add chicken broth, diced tomatoes, apricots, cumin, cinnamon, ginger, salt, and pepper.

4. Bring to a boil, then reduce heat and simmer for 1 hour, or until the lamb is tender.

5. Stir in chopped cilantro before serving.

Nutritional Values (per serving):

- Calories: 350
- Fat: 18g
- Carbohydrates: 22g
- Protein: 25g

Tilapia with Mango Salsa

Ingredients:

- 4 tilapia fillets
- 1 tablespoon olive oil
- Salt and pepper to taste
- 1 ripe mango, diced
- 1/2 red bell pepper, diced
- 1/4 cup red onion, finely chopped (optional if sensitive)
- 1 tablespoon lime juice
- 2 tablespoons chopped fresh cilantro

Directions:

1. Preheat the grill to medium-high heat.

2. Brush tilapia fillets with olive oil and season with salt and pepper.

3. Grill tilapia for 3-4 minutes per side, or until cooked through.

4. In a bowl, combine mango, red bell pepper, red onion (if using), lime juice, and cilantro.

5. Serve grilled tilapia topped with mango salsa.

Nutritional Values (per serving):

- Calories: 220
- Fat: 8g
- Carbohydrates: 14g
- Protein: 25g

Vegetarian Paella

Ingredients:

- 2 tablespoons olive oil
- 1 onion, diced (optional if sensitive)
- 1 red bell pepper, diced
- 1 yellow bell pepper, diced
- 2 cups Arborio rice
- 4 cups low FODMAP vegetable broth
- 1 cup diced tomatoes (no added garlic or onions)
- 1 cup green beans, chopped
- 1 teaspoon smoked paprika
- 1/2 teaspoon saffron threads
- 1 cup frozen peas, thawed
- Salt and pepper to taste

Directions:

1. In a large skillet, heat olive oil over medium heat. Add onion (if using) and bell peppers, cooking until tender.
2. Stir in Arborio rice and cook for 2 minutes.
3. Add vegetable broth, diced tomatoes, green beans, smoked paprika, and saffron threads. Bring to a boil.
4. Reduce heat to low, cover, and simmer for 20-25 minutes, or until the rice is cooked and the liquid is absorbed.
5. Stir in peas and season with salt and pepper before serving.

Nutritional Values (per serving):

- Calories: 300
- Fat: 10g
- Carbohydrates: 50g
- Protein: 6g

Herb Roasted Turkey

Ingredients:

- 1 whole turkey (about 12 pounds)
- 1/4 cup olive oil
- 2 tablespoons chopped fresh rosemary

- 2 tablespoons chopped fresh thyme

- 1 tablespoon chopped fresh sage

- 1 lemon, sliced

- Salt and pepper to taste

Directions:

1. Preheat the oven to 325°F (165°C).

2. In a small bowl, combine olive oil, rosemary, thyme, sage, salt, and pepper.

3. Rub the herb mixture all over the turkey, including under the skin.

4. Stuff the turkey cavity with lemon slices.

5. Place the turkey on a rack in a roasting pan and roast for 3-4 hours, or until the internal temperature reaches 165°F (74°C).

6. Let rest for 20 minutes before carving.

7. Serve warm.

Nutritional Values (per serving):

- Calories: 350

- Fat: 18g

- Carbohydrates: 2g

- Protein: 40g

Low FODMAP Beef Stroganoff

Ingredients:

- 1 pound beef sirloin, sliced into strips

- 2 tablespoons olive oil

- 1 onion, diced (optional if sensitive)

- 1 cup low FODMAP beef broth

- 1/2 cup lactose-free sour cream

- 2 tablespoons Dijon mustard

- 1 tablespoon Worcestershire sauce (ensure it's low FODMAP)

- Salt and pepper to taste

- 8 ounces gluten-free pasta

Directions:

1. In a large skillet, heat olive oil over medium heat. Add beef and cook until browned. Remove and set aside.

2. Add onion (if using) to the skillet and cook until tender.

3. Return beef to the skillet and add beef broth, sour cream, Dijon mustard, Worcestershire sauce, salt, and pepper. Simmer for 10 minutes.

4. Meanwhile, cook gluten-free pasta according to package instructions.

5. Serve beef stroganoff over cooked pasta.

Nutritional Values (per serving):

- Calories: 400

- Fat: 20g

- Carbohydrates: 30g

- Protein: 28g

Stuffed Acorn Squash

Ingredients:

- 2 acorn squashes, halved and seeds removed

- 1 cup cooked quinoa

- 1/2 cup diced tomatoes (no added garlic or onions)

- 1/2 cup chopped spinach

- 1/4 cup crumbled feta cheese

- 1 tablespoon olive oil

- 1 teaspoon dried thyme

- Salt and pepper to taste

Directions:

1. Preheat the oven to 375°F (190°C).

2. Brush acorn squash halves with olive oil and season with salt

and pepper. Place cut side down on a baking sheet and bake for 35-40 minutes, until tender.

3. In a bowl, combine cooked quinoa, diced tomatoes, spinach, feta cheese, thyme, salt, and pepper.

4. Fill each squash half with the quinoa mixture.

5. Return to the oven and bake for an additional 10 minutes.

6. Serve warm.

Nutritional Values (per serving):

- Calories: 250

- Fat: 10g

- Carbohydrates: 35g

- Protein: 6g

Grilled Shrimp Tacos with Pineapple Salsa

Ingredients:

- 1 pound shrimp, peeled and deveined

- 1 tablespoon olive oil

- 1 teaspoon ground cumin

- 1/2 teaspoon smoked paprika

- Salt and pepper to taste

- 8 corn tortillas

- 1 cup diced pineapple
- 1/4 cup red onion, finely chopped (optional if sensitive)
- 1 tablespoon lime juice
- 2 tablespoons chopped fresh cilantro

Directions:

1. Preheat the grill to medium-high heat.
2. Toss shrimp with olive oil, cumin, smoked paprika, salt, and pepper.
3. Grill shrimp for 2-3 minutes per side, or until cooked through.
4. In a bowl, combine pineapple, red onion (if using), lime juice, and cilantro to make the salsa.
5. Warm corn tortillas on the grill.
6. Serve grilled shrimp in tortillas topped with pineapple salsa.

Nutritional Values (per serving):

- Calories: 200
- Fat: 8g
- Carbohydrates: 18g
- Protein: 15g

FODMAP-friendly Chicken Alfredo

Ingredients:

- 2 boneless, skinless chicken breasts, sliced
- 8 ounces gluten-free pasta
- 2 tablespoons olive oil
- 1 cup lactose-free heavy cream
- 1/2 cup grated Parmesan cheese
- 1 teaspoon garlic-infused oil (optional if sensitive)
- Salt and pepper to taste
- Fresh parsley for garnish

Directions:

1. Cook gluten-free pasta according to package instructions. Drain and set aside.
2. In a large skillet, heat olive oil over medium heat. Add chicken and cook until browned and cooked through.
3. Reduce heat to low and stir in lactose-free heavy cream, Parmesan cheese, garlic-infused oil (if using), salt, and pepper. Simmer until the sauce thickens.
4. Toss the cooked pasta with the Alfredo sauce.
5. Serve topped with fresh parsley.

Nutritional Values (per serving):

- Calories: 450
- Fat: 25g
- Carbohydrates: 30g
- Protein: 25g

Baked Trout with Almondine Sauce

Ingredients:

- 4 trout fillets
- 1/4 cup sliced almonds
- 2 tablespoons butter
- 1 tablespoon lemon juice
- 1 tablespoon chopped fresh parsley
- Salt and pepper to taste

Directions:

1. Preheat the oven to 375°F (190°C).
2. Place trout fillets on a baking sheet lined with parchment paper. Season with salt and pepper.
3. Bake for 12-15 minutes, or until the fish is cooked through.
4. In a small skillet, melt butter over medium heat. Add sliced almonds and cook until golden brown. Stir in lemon juice and parsley.
5. Spoon the almondine sauce over the baked trout before serving.

Nutritional Values (per serving):

- Calories: 300
- Fat: 20g
- Carbohydrates: 2g
- Protein: 25g

Vegan Mushroom Risotto

Ingredients:

- 2 tablespoons olive oil
- 1 onion, diced (optional if sensitive)
- 2 cloves garlic, minced (optional if sensitive)
- 1 pound mushrooms, sliced
- 1 cup Arborio rice
- 4 cups low FODMAP vegetable broth, warmed
- 1/4 cup nutritional yeast
- 1 tablespoon chopped fresh thyme
- Salt and pepper to taste

Directions:

1. In a large skillet, heat olive oil over medium heat. Add onion (if using) and garlic (if using), cooking until tender.

2. Add sliced mushrooms and cook until browned.

3. Stir in Arborio rice and cook for 2 minutes.

4. Gradually add warm vegetable broth, one ladle at a time, stirring frequently until absorbed. Continue until the rice is creamy and cooked through.

5. Stir in nutritional yeast, thyme, salt, and pepper.

6. Serve warm.

Nutritional Values (per serving):

- Calories: 300

- Fat: 12g

- Carbohydrates: 40g

- Protein: 8g

BBQ Pulled Pork (Low FODMAP BBQ Sauce)

Ingredients:

- 2 pounds pork shoulder

- 1 cup low FODMAP BBQ sauce

- 1/2 cup apple cider vinegar

- 1/4 cup brown sugar

- 1 tablespoon paprika

- 1 teaspoon salt

- 1/2 teaspoon black pepper

Directions:

1. Preheat the oven to 300°F (150°C).

2. In a bowl, combine BBQ sauce, apple cider vinegar, brown sugar, paprika, salt, and pepper.

3. Place pork shoulder in a roasting pan and pour the sauce mixture over it.

4. Cover with foil and roast for 3-4 hours, or until the pork is tender and easily shredded.

5. Shred the pork with two forks and mix with the sauce.

6. Serve warm.

Nutritional Values (per serving):

- Calories: 350

- Fat: 18g

- Carbohydrates: 20g

- Protein: 25g

Stir-fried Tofu with Low FODMAP Vegetables

Ingredients:

- 1 block firm tofu, drained and cubed
- 2 tablespoons olive oil
- 1 red bell pepper, sliced
- 1 cup snap peas
- 1 zucchini, sliced
- 2 tablespoons low sodium soy sauce (gluten-free)
- 1 tablespoon rice vinegar
- 1 teaspoon sesame oil
- 1 teaspoon grated fresh ginger

Directions:

1. Heat olive oil in a large skillet over medium heat. Add cubed tofu and cook until golden brown on all sides. Remove and set aside.

2. In the same skillet, add bell pepper, snap peas, and zucchini, cooking until tender-crisp.

3. In a small bowl, whisk together soy sauce, rice vinegar, sesame oil, and grated ginger.

4. Return tofu to the skillet and pour the sauce over the vegetables and tofu. Stir to coat and cook for another 2-3 minutes.

5. Serve warm.

Nutritional Values (per serving):

- Calories: 250
- Fat: 15g
- Carbohydrates: 18g
- Protein: 12g

Slow Cooker Chicken and Rice

Ingredients:

- 4 boneless, skinless chicken breasts
- 1 cup uncooked white rice
- 2 cups low FODMAP chicken broth
- 1 cup diced carrots
- 1 cup diced celery (green parts only)
- 1 teaspoon dried thyme
- 1 teaspoon dried oregano
- Salt and pepper to taste

Directions:

1. Place chicken breasts, rice, chicken broth, carrots, celery, thyme, oregano, salt, and pepper in a slow cooker.

2. Cover and cook on low for 4-5 hours, or until the chicken is cooked through and the rice is tender.

3. Shred the chicken and stir to combine.

4. Serve warm.

Nutritional Values (per serving):

- Calories: 300
- Fat: 8g
- Carbohydrates: 30g
- Protein: 25g

Pan-seared Duck Breast with Orange Sauce

Ingredients:

- 2 duck breasts
- Salt and pepper to taste
- 1/2 cup orange juice
- 1 tablespoon honey
- 1 tablespoon balsamic vinegar
- 1 teaspoon grated orange zest

Directions:

1. Score the skin of the duck breasts and season with salt and pepper.

2. Place the duck breasts skin-side down in a cold skillet. Heat over medium heat and cook until the skin is crispy, about 8-10 minutes. Flip and cook for an additional 4-5 minutes, or until desired doneness. Remove and let rest.

3. In the same skillet, combine orange juice, honey, balsamic vinegar, and orange zest. Cook over medium heat until the sauce thickens.

4. Slice the duck breasts and serve with the orange sauce.

Nutritional Values (per serving):

- Calories: 400
- Fat: 28g
- Carbohydrates: 12g
- Protein: 25g

Lasagna with Lactose-Free Ricotta

Ingredients:

- 8 ounces gluten-free lasagna noodles
- 1 pound ground beef
- 2 cups marinara sauce (ensure it's low FODMAP)
- 1 cup lactose-free ricotta cheese
- 1 cup shredded mozzarella cheese
- 1/4 cup grated Parmesan cheese
- 1 egg

- 1 tablespoon chopped fresh basil

- Salt and pepper to taste

Directions:

1. Preheat the oven to 375°F (190°C).

2. Cook gluten-free lasagna noodles according to package instructions. Drain and set aside.

3. In a skillet, cook ground beef over medium heat until browned. Add marinara sauce and simmer for 10 minutes.

4. In a bowl, combine lactose-free ricotta cheese, mozzarella cheese, Parmesan cheese, egg, basil, salt, and pepper.

5. Spread a thin layer of meat sauce in the bottom of a baking dish. Layer with lasagna noodles, ricotta mixture, and meat sauce. Repeat layers, ending with meat sauce on top.

6. Cover with foil and bake for 25 minutes. Remove foil and bake for an additional 10 minutes, until the cheese is melted and bubbly.

7. Let rest for 10 minutes before serving.

Nutritional Values (per serving):

- Calories: 400

- Fat: 20g

- Carbohydrates: 30g

- Protein: 25g

Seafood Paella (Low FODMAP Version)

Ingredients:

- 2 tablespoons olive oil

- 1 red bell pepper, diced

- 1 yellow bell pepper, diced

- 1 cup Arborio rice

- 4 cups low FODMAP seafood broth

- 1/2 cup diced tomatoes (no added garlic or onions)

- 1/2 pound shrimp, peeled and deveined

- 1/2 pound mussels, cleaned

- 1/2 pound clams, cleaned

- 1 teaspoon smoked paprika

- 1/2 teaspoon saffron threads

- 1/4 cup chopped fresh parsley

- Salt and pepper to taste

Directions:

1. In a large skillet, heat olive oil over medium heat. Add bell peppers and cook until tender.

2. Stir in Arborio rice and cook for 2 minutes.

3. Add seafood broth, diced tomatoes, shrimp, mussels, clams, smoked paprika, saffron threads, salt, and pepper. Bring to a boil.

4. Reduce heat to low, cover, and simmer for 20-25 minutes, or until the rice is cooked and the seafood is done.

5. Stir in chopped parsley before serving.

Nutritional Values (per serving):

- Calories: 350
- Fat: 12g
- Carbohydrates: 35g
- Protein: 25g

Thai Green Curry with Chicken

Ingredients:

- 2 tablespoons olive oil
- 1 pound chicken breast, sliced
- 1 cup coconut milk (ensure it's low FODMAP)
- 1 cup green beans, trimmed
- 1 red bell pepper, sliced
- 2 tablespoons green curry paste (ensure it's low FODMAP)
- 1 tablespoon fish sauce
- 1 tablespoon lime juice
- 1/4 cup chopped fresh basil
- Salt and pepper to taste

Directions:

1. In a large skillet, heat olive oil over medium heat. Add chicken and cook until browned.

2. Stir in coconut milk, green beans, bell pepper, green curry paste, fish sauce, and lime juice. Bring to a simmer.

3. Cook for 10-15 minutes, until the vegetables are tender and the chicken is cooked through.

4. Stir in chopped basil and season with salt and pepper.

5. Serve warm.

Nutritional Values (per serving):

- Calories: 350
- Fat: 22g
- Carbohydrates: 12g
- Protein: 25g

Pork Chops with Apples and Cinnamon

Ingredients:

- 4 bone-in pork chops
- 2 tablespoons olive oil
- 2 apples, peeled, cored, and sliced
- 1/4 cup apple cider vinegar
- 1 tablespoon brown sugar
- 1 teaspoon ground cinnamon
- Salt and pepper to taste

Directions:

1. Season pork chops with salt and pepper.
2. In a large skillet, heat olive oil over medium heat. Add pork chops and cook until browned, about 4-5 minutes per side. Remove and set aside.
3. In the same skillet, add apples, apple cider vinegar, brown sugar, and cinnamon. Cook until the apples are tender.
4. Return pork chops to the skillet and cook for an additional 5 minutes, until cooked through.
5. Serve warm with apples and sauce.

Nutritional Values (per serving):

- Calories: 350
- Fat: 18g
- Carbohydrates: 20g
- Protein: 25g

FODMAP-friendly Ratatouille

Ingredients:

- 2 tablespoons olive oil
- 1 eggplant, diced
- 1 zucchini, diced
- 1 yellow squash, diced
- 1 red bell pepper, diced
- 1 can (14.5 ounces) diced tomatoes (no added garlic or onions)
- 1 teaspoon dried thyme
- 1 teaspoon dried basil
- Salt and pepper to taste
- Fresh basil for garnish

Directions:

1. In a large skillet, heat olive oil over medium heat. Add eggplant, zucchini, yellow squash, and bell pepper, cooking until tender.
2. Stir in diced tomatoes, thyme, basil, salt, and pepper. Bring to a simmer.
3. Cook for 20-25 minutes, until the vegetables are soft and the flavors are blended.

4. Garnish with fresh basil before serving.

Nutritional Values (per serving):

- Calories: 180
- Fat: 10g
- Carbohydrates: 20g
- Protein: 3g

Snacks (25 Recipes)

Mixed Berry Compote with Greek Yogurt

Ingredients:

- 2 cups mixed berries (strawberries, blueberries, raspberries)
- 1/4 cup water
- 2 tablespoons maple syrup
- 1 teaspoon lemon juice
- 2 cups lactose-free Greek yogurt

Directions:

1. In a saucepan, combine mixed berries, water, maple syrup, and lemon juice.
2. Bring to a boil, then reduce heat and simmer for 10-15 minutes, until the berries break down and the mixture thickens.
3. Remove from heat and let cool.
4. Serve the compote over lactose-free Greek yogurt.

Nutritional Values (per serving):

- Calories: 150
- Fat: 2g
- Carbohydrates: 25g
- Protein: 8g

Garlic-Free Hummus with Carrot Sticks

Ingredients:

- 1 can chickpeas, rinsed and drained
- 1/4 cup tahini
- 1/4 cup lemon juice
- 1/4 cup water
- 2 tablespoons olive oil
- 1/2 teaspoon ground cumin
- Salt and pepper to taste
- Carrot sticks for serving

Directions:

1. In a food processor, combine chickpeas, tahini, lemon juice, water, olive oil, cumin, salt, and pepper.
2. Blend until smooth, adding more water if needed for desired consistency.
3. Serve with carrot sticks.

Nutritional Values (per serving):

- Calories: 180
- Fat: 10g
- Carbohydrates: 18g

- Protein: 6g

Peanut Butter Banana Smoothie

Ingredients:

- 1 ripe banana
- 2 tablespoons peanut butter
- 1 cup lactose-free milk
- 1/2 cup ice
- 1 teaspoon honey (optional)

Directions:

1. Combine banana, peanut butter, lactose-free milk, ice, and honey (if using) in a blender.
2. Blend until smooth.
3. Pour into a glass and serve immediately.

Nutritional Values (per serving):

- Calories: 250
- Fat: 12g
- Carbohydrates: 30g
- Protein: 10g

Lactose-Free Cheese and Rice Crackers

Ingredients:

- 1/4 cup lactose-free cheese, cubed

- 1 cup rice crackers

Directions:

1. Arrange lactose-free cheese cubes on a plate.
2. Serve with rice crackers.

Nutritional Values (per serving):

- Calories: 150
- Fat: 7g
- Carbohydrates: 18g
- Protein: 5g

Roasted Chickpeas with Sea Salt

Ingredients:

- 1 can chickpeas, rinsed and drained
- 1 tablespoon olive oil
- 1/2 teaspoon sea salt

Directions:

1. Preheat the oven to 400°F (200°C).
2. Toss chickpeas with olive oil and sea salt.
3. Spread chickpeas on a baking sheet and roast for 25-30 minutes, until crispy.
4. Let cool before serving.

Nutritional Values (per serving):

- Calories: 150
- Fat: 7g
- Carbohydrates: 18g
- Protein: 5g

Pineapple and Cottage Cheese

Ingredients:

- 1 cup fresh pineapple, diced
- 1/2 cup lactose-free cottage cheese

Directions:

1. In a bowl, combine diced pineapple and lactose-free cottage cheese.
2. Serve immediately.

Nutritional Values (per serving):

- Calories: 150
- Fat: 2g
- Carbohydrates: 25g
- Protein: 10g

Cucumber and Dill Dip

Ingredients:

- 1 cup lactose-free Greek yogurt
- 1/2 cucumber, grated and drained
- 1 tablespoon fresh dill, chopped
- 1 tablespoon lemon juice
- Salt and pepper to taste

Directions:

1. In a bowl, combine lactose-free Greek yogurt, grated cucumber, dill, lemon juice, salt, and pepper.
2. Mix well and chill for 30 minutes before serving.
3. Serve with vegetable sticks or gluten-free crackers.

Nutritional Values (per serving):

- Calories: 80
- Fat: 2g
- Carbohydrates: 10g
- Protein: 6g

Stuffed Mini Peppers

Ingredients:

- 12 mini bell peppers
- 1/2 cup lactose-free cream cheese
- 1/4 cup crumbled feta cheese
- 2 tablespoons chopped fresh parsley
- Salt and pepper to taste

Directions:

1. Cut the tops off the mini bell peppers and remove the seeds.

2. In a bowl, combine lactose-free cream cheese, crumbled feta, parsley, salt, and pepper.

3. Fill each mini pepper with the cheese mixture.

4. Serve immediately or chill until ready to serve.

Nutritional Values (per serving):

- Calories: 150
- Fat: 10g
- Carbohydrates: 10g
- Protein: 5g

Gluten-Free Pretzels with Cheddar

Ingredients:

- 1 cup gluten-free pretzels
- 1/4 cup lactose-free cheddar cheese, cubed

Directions:

1. Arrange gluten-free pretzels on a plate.

2. Serve with cubed lactose-free cheddar cheese.

Nutritional Values (per serving):

- Calories: 180
- Fat: 8g
- Carbohydrates: 20g
- Protein: 6g

Low FODMAP Trail Mix

Ingredients:

- 1/4 cup almonds
- 1/4 cup walnuts
- 1/4 cup pumpkin seeds
- 1/4 cup dried cranberries (ensure they are low FODMAP)

Directions:

1. In a bowl, combine almonds, walnuts, pumpkin seeds, and dried cranberries.

2. Mix well and store in an airtight container.

Nutritional Values (per serving):

- Calories: 200
- Fat: 15g
- Carbohydrates: 14g
- Protein: 5g

Coconut Macaroons

Ingredients:

- 2 cups shredded coconut
- 1/2 cup sugar
- 2 large egg whites

- 1 teaspoon vanilla extract

Directions:

1. Preheat the oven to 325°F (165°C) and line a baking sheet with parchment paper.

2. In a bowl, combine shredded coconut, sugar, egg whites, and vanilla extract.

3. Drop spoonfuls of the mixture onto the prepared baking sheet.

4. Bake for 20-25 minutes, until golden brown.

5. Let cool before serving.

Nutritional Values (per serving):

- Calories: 150
- Fat: 8g
- Carbohydrates: 18g
- Protein: 2g

Spiced Popcorn

Ingredients:

- 1/4 cup popcorn kernels
- 2 tablespoons olive oil
- 1/2 teaspoon ground cumin
- 1/2 teaspoon smoked paprika
- 1/4 teaspoon salt

Directions:

1. In a large pot, heat olive oil over medium heat. Add popcorn kernels and cover with a lid.

2. Shake the pot occasionally until the popping slows down.

3. Remove from heat and transfer popcorn to a large bowl.

4. Sprinkle with cumin, smoked paprika, and salt. Toss to coat evenly.

Nutritional Values (per serving):

- Calories: 100
- Fat: 7g
- Carbohydrates: 10g
- Protein: 2g

Baked Kale Chips

Ingredients:

- 1 bunch kale, washed and dried
- 1 tablespoon olive oil
- 1/2 teaspoon sea salt

Directions:

1. Preheat the oven to 350°F (175°C) and line a baking sheet with parchment paper.

2. Remove the kale leaves from the stems and tear into bite-sized pieces.

3. In a bowl, toss kale with olive oil and sea salt.

4. Spread kale on the baking sheet in a single layer.

5. Bake for 10-15 minutes, until crispy.

6. Let cool before serving.

Nutritional Values (per serving):

- Calories: 50
- Fat: 3g
- Carbohydrates: 5g
- Protein: 2g

Mashed Avocado on Rice Cakes

Ingredients:

- 1 ripe avocado
- 1 tablespoon lemon juice
- Salt and pepper to taste
- 4 rice cakes

Directions:

1. In a bowl, mash the avocado with lemon juice, salt, and pepper.

2. Spread the mashed avocado on rice cakes.

3. Serve immediately.

Nutritional Values (per serving):

- Calories: 150
- Fat: 10g
- Carbohydrates: 15g
- Protein: 2g

Raspberry Sorbet

Ingredients:

- 2 cups fresh raspberries
- 1/2 cup water
- 1/4 cup sugar
- 1 tablespoon lemon juice

Directions:

1. In a blender, combine raspberries, water, sugar, and lemon juice.

2. Blend until smooth.

3. Pour the mixture into a shallow container and freeze for at least 4 hours, stirring occasionally.

4. Serve frozen.

Nutritional Values (per serving):

- Calories: 80
- Fat: 0g
- Carbohydrates: 20g
- Protein: 1g

Parmesan Crisps

Ingredients:

- 1 cup grated Parmesan cheese

Directions:

1. Preheat the oven to 400°F (200°C) and line a baking sheet with parchment paper.

2. Spoon tablespoons of grated Parmesan cheese onto the baking sheet, flattening each mound slightly.

3. Bake for 5-7 minutes, until golden and crispy.

4. Let cool before serving.

Nutritional Values (per serving):

- Calories: 100
- Fat: 7g
- Carbohydrates: 1g
- Protein: 9g

Baked Apple Chips

Ingredients:

- 2 apples, thinly sliced
- 1 teaspoon ground cinnamon

Directions:

1. Preheat the oven to 225°F (110°C) and line a baking sheet with parchment paper.

2. Arrange apple slices on the baking sheet in a single layer.

3. Sprinkle with ground cinnamon.

4. Bake for 1.5-2 hours, until the apples are dried and crispy.

5. Let cool before serving.

Nutritional Values (per serving):

- Calories: 80
- Fat: 0g
- Carbohydrates: 21g
- Protein: 0g

Chocolate-dipped Strawberries (Dark Chocolate)

Ingredients:

- 1 cup dark chocolate chips
- 1 tablespoon coconut oil
- 1 pint fresh strawberries

Directions:

1. In a microwave-safe bowl, combine dark chocolate chips and coconut oil. Microwave in 30-second intervals, stirring between each, until melted and smooth.

2. Dip each strawberry into the melted chocolate, letting the excess drip off.

3. Place the dipped strawberries on a parchment-lined baking sheet.

4. Refrigerate for 30 minutes, until the chocolate is set.

Nutritional Values (per serving):

- Calories: 120
- Fat: 8g
- Carbohydrates: 15g
- Protein: 1g

Rice Pudding with Vanilla

Ingredients:

- 1/2 cup Arborio rice
- 2 cups lactose-free milk
- 1/4 cup sugar
- 1 teaspoon vanilla extract
- 1/4 teaspoon ground cinnamon

Directions:

1. In a saucepan, combine Arborio rice, lactose-free milk, and sugar. Bring to a boil.

2. Reduce heat and simmer, stirring frequently, until the rice is tender and the mixture is creamy, about 20-25 minutes.

3. Stir in vanilla extract and ground cinnamon.

4. Serve warm or chilled.

Nutritional Values (per serving):

- Calories: 200
- Fat: 4g
- Carbohydrates: 35g
- Protein: 6g

Peanut Butter and Oatmeal Cookies

Ingredients:

- 1 cup rolled oats
- 1/2 cup peanut butter
- 1/4 cup maple syrup
- 1/4 cup lactose-free milk
- 1 teaspoon vanilla extract
- 1/2 teaspoon baking soda
- 1/4 teaspoon salt

Directions:

1. Preheat the oven to 350°F (175°C) and line a baking sheet with parchment paper.

2. In a bowl, combine rolled oats, peanut butter, maple syrup, lactose-free milk, vanilla extract, baking soda, and salt.

3. Drop spoon fuls of dough onto the prepared baking sheet.

4. Bake for 10-12 minutes, until golden brown.

5. Let cool before serving.

Nutritional Values (per serving):

- Calories: 150
- Fat: 8g
- Carbohydrates: 15g
- Protein: 4g

Roasted Nuts with Rosemary

Ingredients:

- 2 cups mixed nuts (almonds, walnuts, pecans)
- 2 tablespoons olive oil
- 1 tablespoon chopped fresh rosemary
- 1/2 teaspoon sea salt

Directions:

1. Preheat the oven to 350°F (175°C) and line a baking sheet with parchment paper.
2. In a bowl, toss mixed nuts with olive oil, rosemary, and sea salt.
3. Spread nuts on the baking sheet in a single layer.
4. Roast for 15-20 minutes, stirring occasionally, until golden and fragrant.
5. Let cool before serving.

Nutritional Values (per serving):

- Calories: 200
- Fat: 18g
- Carbohydrates: 6g
- Protein: 5g

Lemon Bars (Gluten-Free)

Ingredients:

- 1 cup gluten-free flour
- 1/2 cup butter, melted
- 1/4 cup sugar
- 3 large eggs
- 1 cup sugar
- 1/4 cup gluten-free flour
- 1/2 cup lemon juice
- 1 tablespoon lemon zest

Directions:

1. Preheat the oven to 350°F (175°C) and line an 8x8-inch baking dish with parchment paper.
2. In a bowl, combine 1 cup gluten-free flour, melted butter, and 1/4 cup sugar. Press into the bottom of the prepared baking dish.
3. Bake for 15-20 minutes, until lightly golden.

4. In another bowl, whisk together eggs, 1 cup sugar, 1/4 cup gluten-free flour, lemon juice, and lemon zest.

5. Pour the lemon mixture over the baked crust.

6. Bake for an additional 20-25 minutes, until set.

7. Let cool before cutting into squares.

Nutritional Values (per serving):

- Calories: 200

- Fat: 10g

- Carbohydrates: 28g

- Protein: 3g

FODMAP-friendly Pita Chips

Ingredients:

- 4 gluten-free pita breads

- 2 tablespoons olive oil

- 1 teaspoon dried oregano

- 1/2 teaspoon sea salt

Directions:

1. Preheat the oven to 375°F (190°C) and line a baking sheet with parchment paper.

2. Cut gluten-free pita breads into wedges.

3. In a bowl, toss pita wedges with olive oil, oregano, and sea salt.

4. Spread pita wedges on the baking sheet in a single layer.

5. Bake for 10-15 minutes, until crispy.

6. Let cool before serving.

Nutritional Values (per serving):

- Calories: 150

- Fat: 6g

- Carbohydrates: 20g

- Protein: 2g

Mozzarella Sticks (Lactose-Free)

Ingredients:

- 8 sticks lactose-free mozzarella cheese

- 1/2 cup gluten-free flour

- 2 large eggs, beaten

- 1 cup gluten-free breadcrumbs

- 1/2 teaspoon dried oregano

- 1/2 teaspoon dried basil

- Olive oil for frying

Directions:

1. Cut each mozzarella stick in half.

2. Dredge each piece in gluten-free flour, then dip in beaten eggs, and coat with gluten-free breadcrumbs mixed with oregano and basil.

3. Heat olive oil in a skillet over medium heat.

4. Fry the mozzarella sticks until golden brown and crispy.

5. Drain on paper towels before serving.

Nutritional Values (per serving):

- Calories: 250
- Fat: 15g
- Carbohydrates: 15g
- Protein: 10g

Prosciutto-wrapped Melon

Ingredients:

- 1 cantaloupe, cut into wedges
- 8 slices prosciutto, halved

Directions:

1. Wrap each cantaloupe wedge with a piece of prosciutto.

2. Serve immediately.

Nutritional Values (per serving):

- Calories: 70
- Fat: 3g
- Carbohydrates: 8g
- Protein: 3g

CHAPTER 4

58-DAY MEAL PLAN

Creating a sustainable and enjoyable low FODMAP diet can be a rewarding journey, especially when you have a structured plan to guide you. This 58-day meal plan is designed to simplify your daily meal preparation while ensuring you enjoy a variety of delicious, gut-friendly foods. By following this plan, you will not only manage your IBS symptoms more effectively but also discover a wealth of new recipes that bring both comfort and nourishment. Each day's meals are carefully curated to balance flavors, textures, and nutritional needs, making it easier to stick to the diet without feeling deprived. Whether you're new to the low FODMAP diet or looking for fresh ideas to revitalize your routine, this plan provides a clear, step-by-step approach to maintaining your digestive health. Dive in, explore the culinary possibilities, and experience the positive changes that come with a well-structured meal plan tailored to your needs.

58-Day Meal Plan

Week 1

Day 1

- Breakfast: Sunrise Smoothie with Banana and Strawberry

- Snack: Roasted Chickpeas with Sea Salt

- Lunch: Grilled Chicken Salad with Low FODMAP Vinaigrette

- Snack: Mixed Berry Compote with Greek Yogurt

- Dinner: Maple-Glazed Pork Tenderloin with a side of steamed green beans

Day 2

- Breakfast: Blueberry Infused Quinoa Porridge
- Snack: Lactose-Free Cheese and Rice Crackers
- Lunch: Turkey and Swiss Cheese Wrap
- Snack: Cucumber and Dill Dip with gluten-free crackers
- Dinner: Baked Cod with Olive Tapenade and a side of roasted carrots

Day 3

- Breakfast: Spinach and Feta Omelet
- Snack: Peanut Butter Banana Smoothie
- Lunch: Quinoa Tabbouleh with Cucumbers
- Snack: Pineapple and Cottage Cheese
- Dinner: Spaghetti Squash with Tomato Sauce

Day 4

- Breakfast: Cinnamon Buckwheat Pancakes
- Snack: Garlic-Free Hummus with Carrot Sticks
- Lunch: Low FODMAP Minestrone Soup
- Snack: Mashed Avocado on Rice Cakes
- Dinner: Grilled Steak with Low FODMAP Chimichurri and a side of roasted potatoes

Day 5

- Breakfast: Maple-Glazed Chicken Sausage Patties
- Snack: Baked Kale Chips
- Lunch: Baked Salmon with Herb Crust and a side salad
- Snack: Gluten-Free Pretzels with Cheddar
- Dinner: Lemon Garlic Roasted Chicken with sautéed spinach

Day 6

- Breakfast: Low FODMAP Muesli with Oats and Seeds

- Snack: Spiced Popcorn
- Lunch: Rice Paper Rolls with Shrimp
- Snack: Stuffed Mini Peppers
- Dinner: Eggplant Parmesan (Gluten-Free) with a side of steamed broccoli

Day 7

- Breakfast: Lactose-Free Yogurt Parfait with Kiwi
- Snack: Low FODMAP Trail Mix
- Lunch: Greek Salad with Feta and Olives
- Snack: Chocolate-dipped Strawberries (Dark Chocolate)
- Dinner: Moroccan Lamb Stew with quinoa

Week 2

Day 8

- Breakfast: Sweet Potato and Bacon Hash
- Snack: Coconut Macaroons
- Lunch: Sourdough Grilled Cheese with Spinach

- Snack: Baked Apple Chips
- Dinner: Tilapia with Mango Salsa and a side of steamed rice

Day 9

- Breakfast: Raspberry Chia Pudding
- Snack: Parmesan Crisps
- Lunch: Tuna Salad Stuffed Bell Peppers
- Snack: Roasted Nuts with Rosemary
- Dinner: Vegetarian Paella

Day 10

- Breakfast: Spiced Pumpkin Waffles
- Snack: Mixed Berry Compote with Greek Yogurt
- Lunch: Vegetable Stir-fry with Ginger Sauce
- Snack: Peanut Butter and Oatmeal Cookies
- Dinner: Herb Roasted Turkey with roasted sweet potatoes

Day 11

- Breakfast: Scrambled Tofu with Bell Peppers
- Snack: Garlic-Free Hummus with Carrot Sticks
- Lunch: Chicken Caesar Salad (Lactose-Free Dressing)
- Snack: Pineapple and Cottage Cheese
- Dinner: Low FODMAP Beef Stroganoff with gluten-free pasta

Day 12

- Breakfast: Ginger Pear Overnight Oats
- Snack: Spiced Popcorn
- Lunch: FODMAP-friendly Falafel Bowls
- Snack: Lemon Bars (Gluten-Free)
- Dinner: Stuffed Acorn Squash

Day 13

- Breakfast: FODMAP-friendly Eggs Benedict
- Snack: Lactose-Free Cheese and Rice Crackers
- Lunch: Turkey Meatballs with Gluten-Free Pasta
- Snack: Mashed Avocado on Rice Cakes
- Dinner: Grilled Shrimp Tacos with Pineapple Salsa

Day 14

- Breakfast: Turkey and Egg Breakfast Burrito
- Snack: Roasted Chickpeas with Sea Salt
- Lunch: Egg Salad on Gluten-Free Bread
- Snack: Cucumber and Dill Dip with gluten-free crackers
- Dinner: FODMAP-friendly Chicken Alfredo

Week 3

Day 15

- Breakfast: Green Smoothie Bowl
- Snack: Baked Kale Chips
- Lunch: Roasted Vegetable and Quinoa Salad

- Snack: Coconut Macaroons
- Dinner: Baked Trout with Almondine Sauce and a side of sautéed green beans

Day 16

- Breakfast: Strawberry Almond Muffins
- Snack: Parmesan Crisps
- Lunch: Beef and Spinach Stuffed Peppers
- Snack: Gluten-Free Pretzels with Cheddar
- Dinner: Vegan Mushroom Risotto

Day 17

- Breakfast: Baked Oatmeal with Blueberries
- Snack: Roasted Nuts with Rosemary
- Lunch: Caprese Salad with Balsamic Glaze
- Snack: Low FODMAP Trail Mix
- Dinner: BBQ Pulled Pork (Low FODMAP BBQ Sauce) with a side of coleslaw

Day 18

- Breakfast: Quinoa Breakfast Bars
- Snack: Chocolate-dipped Strawberries (Dark Chocolate)
- Lunch: Lemon Herb Chicken Breast with a side of roasted carrots
- Snack: Baked Apple Chips
- Dinner: Stir-fried Tofu with Low FODMAP Vegetables

Day 19

- Breakfast: Lactose-Free Cottage Cheese with Pineapple
- Snack: Spiced Popcorn
- Lunch: Lentil Soup with Carrots and Celery
- Snack: Peanut Butter and Oatmeal Cookies
- Dinner: Slow Cooker Chicken and Rice

Day 20

- Breakfast: Sourdough French Toast with Maple Syrup
- Snack: Garlic-Free Hummus with Carrot Sticks
- Lunch: Avocado and Shrimp Rice Bowl
- Snack: Mashed Avocado on Rice Cakes
- Dinner: Pan-seared Duck Breast with Orange Sauce and a side of roasted Brussels sprouts

Day 21

- Breakfast: Poached Eggs over Polenta
- Snack: Mixed Berry Compote with Greek Yogurt
- Lunch: Baked Haddock with Lemon and Dill and a side of steamed asparagus
- Snack: Coconut Macaroons
- Dinner: Lasagna with Lactose-Free Ricotta

Week 4

Day 22

- Breakfast: Rice Cereal with Cinnamon Apples
- Snack: Roasted Chickpeas with Sea Salt
- Lunch: Seafood Paella (Low FODMAP Version)
- Snack: Gluten-Free Pretzels with Cheddar
- Dinner: Thai Green Curry with Chicken and a side of steamed rice

Day 23

- Breakfast: Turkey Sausage and Bell Pepper Skillet
- Snack: Parmesan Crisps
- Lunch: Turkey and Swiss Cheese Wrap
- Snack: Spiced Popcorn
- Dinner: Pork Chops with Apples and Cinnamon and a side of mashed potatoes

Day 24

- Breakfast: Oat and Banana Pancakes

- Snack: Lactose-Free Cheese and Rice Crackers
- Lunch: Grilled Chicken Salad with Low FODMAP Vinaigrette
- Snack: Cucumber and Dill Dip with gluten-free crackers
- Dinner: FODMAP-friendly Ratatouille

Day 25

- Breakfast: Zucchini and Carrot Fritters
- Snack: Peanut Butter Banana Smoothie
- Lunch: Low FODMAP Minestrone Soup
- Snack: Mashed Avocado on Rice Cakes
- Dinner: Maple-Glazed Pork Tenderloin with a side of roasted Brussels sprouts

Day 26

- Breakfast: Sunrise Smoothie with Banana and Strawberry

- Snack: Roasted Nuts with Rosemary
- Lunch: Baked Salmon with Herb Crust and a side salad
- Snack: Lemon Bars (Gluten-Free)
- Dinner: Spaghetti Squash with Tomato Sauce

Day 27

- Breakfast: Blueberry Infused Quinoa Porridge
- Snack: Mixed Berry Compote with Greek Yogurt
- Lunch: Tuna Salad Stuffed Bell Peppers
- Snack: Garlic-Free Hummus with Carrot Sticks
- Dinner: Grilled Steak with Low FODMAP Chimichurri and a side of roasted potatoes

Day 28

- Breakfast: Spinach and Feta Omelet
- Snack: Spiced Popcorn

- Lunch: Quinoa Tabbouleh with Cucumbers
- Snack: Gluten-Free Pretzels with Cheddar
- Dinner: Lemon Garlic Roasted Chicken with sautéed spinach

Week 5

Day 29

- Breakfast: Cinnamon Buckwheat Pancakes
- Snack: Roasted Chickpeas with Sea Salt
- Lunch: Rice Paper Rolls with Shrimp
- Snack: Peanut Butter and Oatmeal Cookies
- Dinner: Eggplant Parmesan (Gluten-Free) with a side of steamed broccoli

Day 30

- Breakfast: Maple-Glazed Chicken Sausage Patties
- Snack: Mixed Berry Compote with Greek Yogurt

- Lunch: Greek Salad with Feta and Olives
- Snack: Mashed Avocado on Rice Cakes
- Dinner: Moroccan Lamb Stew with quinoa

Day 31

- Breakfast: Low FODMAP Muesli with Oats and Seeds
- Snack: Coconut Macaroons
- Lunch: Sourdough Grilled Cheese with Spinach
- Snack: Parmesan Crisps
- Dinner: Tilapia with Mango Salsa and a side of steamed rice

Day 32

- Breakfast: Lactose-Free Yogurt Parfait with Kiwi
- Snack: Spiced Popcorn
- Lunch: Vegetable Stir-fry with Ginger Sauce
- Snack: Garlic-Free Hummus with Carrot Sticks
- Dinner: Herb Roasted Turkey with roasted sweet potatoes

Day 33

- Breakfast: Sweet Potato and Bacon Hash
- Snack: Roasted Nuts with Rosemary
- Lunch: Chicken Caesar Salad (Lactose-Free Dressing)
- Snack: Mixed Berry Compote with Greek Yogurt
- Dinner: Low FODMAP Beef Stroganoff with gluten-free pasta

Day 34

- Breakfast: Raspberry Chia Pudding
- Snack: Lemon Bars (Gluten-Free)
- Lunch: FODMAP-friendly Falafel Bowls
- Snack: Gluten-Free Pretzels with Cheddar
- Dinner: Stuffed Acorn Squash

Day 35

- Breakfast: Spiced Pumpkin Waffles
- Snack: Peanut Butter Banana Smoothie
- Lunch: Turkey Meatballs with Gluten-Free Pasta
- Snack: Baked Apple Chips
- Dinner: Grilled Shrimp Tacos with Pineapple Salsa

Week 6

Day 36

- Breakfast: Scrambled Tofu with Bell Peppers
- Snack: Spiced Popcorn
- Lunch: Egg Salad on Gluten-Free Bread
- Snack: Coconut Macaroons
- Dinner: FODMAP-friendly Chicken Alfredo

Day 37

- Breakfast: Ginger Pear Overnight Oats
- Snack: Roasted Chickpeas with Sea Salt

- Lunch: Roasted Vegetable and Quinoa Salad
- Snack: Garlic-Free Hummus with Carrot Sticks
- Dinner: Baked Trout with Almondine Sauce and a side of sautéed green beans

Day 38

- Breakfast: FODMAP-friendly Eggs Benedict
- Snack: Mixed Berry Compote with Greek Yogurt
- Lunch: Beef and Spinach Stuffed Peppers
- Snack: Mashed Avocado on Rice Cakes
- Dinner: Vegan Mushroom Risotto

Day 39

- Breakfast: Turkey and Egg Breakfast Burrito
- Snack: Roasted Nuts with Rosemary
- Lunch: Caprese Salad with Balsamic Glaze
- Snack: Spiced Popcorn

- Dinner: BBQ Pulled Pork (Low FODMAP BBQ Sauce) with a side of coleslaw

Day 40

- Breakfast: Green Smoothie Bowl
- Snack: Lemon Bars (Gluten-Free)
- Lunch: Lemon Herb Chicken Breast with a side of roasted carrots
- Snack: Peanut Butter and Oatmeal Cookies
- Dinner: Stir-fried Tofu with Low FODMAP Vegetables

Day 41

- Breakfast: Strawberry Almond Muffins
- Snack: Mixed Berry Compote with Greek Yogurt
- Lunch: Lentil Soup with Carrots and Celery
- Snack: Parmesan Crisps

- Dinner: Slow Cooker Chicken and Rice

Day 42

- Breakfast: Baked Oatmeal with Blueberries
- Snack: Garlic-Free Hummus with Carrot Sticks
- Lunch: Avocado and Shrimp Rice Bowl
- Snack: Gluten-Free Pretzels with Cheddar
- Dinner: Pan-seared Duck Breast with Orange Sauce and a side of roasted Brussels sprouts

Week 7

Day 43

- Breakfast: Quinoa Breakfast Bars
- Snack: Roasted Chickpeas with Sea Salt
- Lunch: Baked Haddock with Lemon and Dill and a side of steamed asparagus
- Snack: Baked Apple Chips
- Dinner: Lasagna with Lactose-Free Ricotta

Day 44

- Breakfast: Lactose-Free Cottage Cheese with Pineapple
- Snack: Spiced Popcorn
- Lunch: Seafood Paella (Low FODMAP Version)
- Snack: Peanut Butter and Oatmeal Cookies
- Dinner: Thai Green Curry with Chicken and a side of steamed rice

Day 45

- Breakfast: Sourdough French Toast with Maple Syrup
- Snack: Mixed Berry Compote with Greek Yogurt
- Lunch: Turkey and Swiss Cheese Wrap
- Snack: Coconut Macaroons
- Dinner: Pork Chops with Apples and Cinnamon and a side of mashed potatoes

Day 46

- Breakfast: Poached Eggs over Polenta
- Snack: Roasted Nuts with Rosemary
- Lunch: Grilled Chicken Salad with Low FODMAP Vinaigrette
- Snack: Spiced Popcorn
- Dinner: FODMAP-friendly Ratatouille

Day 47

- Breakfast: Rice Cereal with Cinnamon Apples
- Snack: Garlic-Free Hummus with Carrot Sticks
- Lunch: Low FODMAP Minestrone Soup
- Snack: Mixed Berry Compote with Greek Yogurt
- Dinner: Maple-Glazed Pork Tenderloin with a side of roasted Brussels sprouts

Day 48

- Breakfast: Turkey Sausage and Bell Pepper Skillet
- Snack: Parmesan Crisps
- Lunch: Baked Salmon with Herb Crust and a side salad
- Snack: Mashed Avocado on Rice Cakes
- Dinner: Spaghetti Squash with Tomato Sauce

Day 49

- Breakfast: Oat and Banana Pancakes
- Snack: Roasted Chickpeas with Sea Salt
- Lunch: Tuna Salad Stuffed Bell Peppers
- Snack: Gluten-Free Pretzels with Cheddar
- Dinner: Grilled Steak with Low FODMAP Chimichurri and a side of roasted potatoes

Week 8

Day 50

- Breakfast: Zucchini and Carrot Fritters
- Snack: Mixed Berry Compote with Greek Yogurt

- Lunch: Quinoa Tabbouleh with Cucumbers
- Snack: Garlic-Free Hummus with Carrot Sticks
- Dinner: Lemon Garlic Roasted Chicken with sautéed spinach

Day 51

- Breakfast: Sunrise Smoothie with Banana and Strawberry
- Snack: Roasted Nuts with Rosemary
- Lunch: Rice Paper Rolls with Shrimp
- Snack: Coconut Macaroons
- Dinner: Eggplant Parmesan (Gluten-Free) with a side of steamed broccoli

Day 52

- Breakfast: Blueberry Infused Quinoa Porridge
- Snack: Lemon Bars (Gluten-Free)
- Lunch: Greek Salad with Feta and Olives
- Snack: Spiced Popcorn

- Dinner: Moroccan Lamb Stew with quinoa

Day 53

- Breakfast: Spinach and Feta Omelet
- Snack: Garlic-Free Hummus with Carrot Sticks
- Lunch: Sourdough Grilled Cheese with Spinach
- Snack: Mixed Berry Compote with Greek Yogurt
- Dinner: Tilapia with Mango Salsa and a side of steamed rice

Day 54

- Breakfast: Cinnamon Buckwheat Pancakes
- Snack: Peanut Butter and Oatmeal Cookies
- Lunch: Vegetable Stir-fry with Ginger Sauce
- Snack: Roasted Chickpeas with Sea Salt
- Dinner: Herb Roasted Turkey with roasted sweet potatoes

Day 55

- Breakfast: Maple-Glazed Chicken Sausage Patties
- Snack: Parmesan Crisps
- Lunch: Chicken Caesar Salad (Lactose-Free Dressing)
- Snack: Mashed Avocado on Rice Cakes
- Dinner: Low FODMAP Beef Stroganoff with gluten-free pasta

Day 56

- Breakfast: Low FODMAP Muesli with Oats and Seeds
- Snack: Spiced Popcorn
- Lunch: FODMAP-friendly Falafel Bowls
- Snack: Baked Apple Chips
- Dinner: Stuffed Acorn Squash

Day 57

- Breakfast: Lactose-Free Yogurt Parfait with Kiwi
- Snack: Roasted Nuts with Rosemary
- Lunch: Turkey Meatballs with Gluten-Free Pasta
- Snack: Mixed Berry Compote with Greek Yogurt
- Dinner: Grilled Shrimp Tacos with Pineapple Salsa

Day 58

- Breakfast: Sweet Potato and Bacon Hash
- Snack: Coconut Macaroons
- Lunch: Egg Salad on Gluten-Free Bread
- Snack: Lemon Bars (Gluten-Free)
- Dinner: FODMAP-friendly Chicken Alfredo

Scan the QR Code and access your 3 bonuses in digital format

🔥 **Bonus 1: Dining Out Low FODMAP Guide**

🔥 **Bonus 2: Stress Management for IBS Relief**

🔥 **Bonus 3: The Ultimate Low FODMAP Shopping List**

Made in the USA
Las Vegas, NV
18 October 2024

97056455R00057